Film/Video-Based Therapy and Trauma

This book uses film/video-based therapy to help build resilience in facing personal, communal, national, and global trauma triggers.

Offering a rich and diverse range of perspectives on trauma, this volume advocates positive social change using therapeutic techniques in filmmaking as well as film/video-based therapy, in conjunction with expressive art therapies such as drama, dance, music, painting, drawing, and more. Chapter authors address issues in one's home, community, country, and the world using integrative medicine and advocacy using film/video-based therapy and digital storytelling. The book highlights psychological trauma and how one can cope with the overwhelming triggers in today's world. It represents an articulate and comprehensive analysis of the ways in which traumatic human experience impacts, and is modified by, film and video media. Representing a rich and diverse range of perspectives on trauma through the lens of a camera, the authors document important examples of moments in which artistic expression becomes human resilience.

Demonstrating how the language of film can facilitate watching, processing, and discussing images of trauma in therapy, in the home, in the community, and in the world, this volume will be of interest to educators and mental health practitioners with an interest in advancing psychotherapy and counseling techniques.

Joshua L. Cohen is clinically trained as a researcher from Pacifica Graduate Institute and Walden University and is the founder and CEO of Media Psychology Consultants and Your Digital Storytelling Project in Los Angeles, USA.

Advances in Mental Health Research series
Books in this series:

Film/Video-Based Therapy and Trauma

Research and Practice

Edited by Joshua L. Cohen

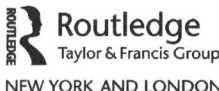
Routledge
Taylor & Francis Group

NEW YORK AND LONDON

First published 2023
by Routledge
605 Third Avenue, New York, NY 10158

and by Routledge
4 Park Square, Milton Park, Abingdon, Oxon, OX14 4RN

Routledge is an imprint of the Taylor & Francis Group, an informa business

© 2023 Taylor & Francis

The right of Joshua L. Cohen to be identified as the author of the editorial material, and of the authors for their individual chapters, has been asserted in accordance with sections 77 and 78 of the Copyright, Designs and Patents Act 1988.

ISBN: 978-1-138-65540-9 (hbk)
ISBN: 978-1-032-40576-6 (pbk)
ISBN: 978-1-315-62250-7 (ebk)

DOI: 10.4324/9781315622507

Typeset in Sabon
by SPi Technologies India Pvt Ltd (Straive)

Contents

Illustrations

Figures

Tables

Contributors

Brooke Campbell, MA, is the founder and director of Creative Kinections, Creative Kinections Institute, and The Mighty Oak. She holds a master's degree from New York University in Drama Therapy and a certificate in Social Impact Strategy from the University of Pennsylvania within their School of Social Policy and Practice. She is a licensed creative arts therapist, board-certified trainer of drama therapy, and a registered drama therapist with 17 years of experience working with diverse populations. Through her work with Creative Kinections, Brooke has formed partnerships with schools, non profit organizations, hospitals, domestic violence agencies, and addiction centers. Brooke has taught at the University of Pennsylvania and guest lectures at various universities such as New York University and Rutgers University, and she presents nationally. Brooke received the NJ Favorite Kids' Doc award for psychotherapy from 2013 to 2019 and received the Women's Excellence award in 2018 for Children's Advocacy. She received the volunteer service award in 2018 from the North American Drama Therapy Association for her work advocating for a drama therapy bill.

Dr. Joshua L. Cohen, PhD, is clinically trained as a researcher from Pacifica Graduate Institute and Walden University. He has experience as a film/video editor, which includes "A" list work in Hollywood with significant people in the film world. He is a media psychologist and CEO of Your Digital Storytelling Project and Media Psychology Consultants and staff with the Kolnoam school of video therapy. Dr. Cohen's clinical experience involves working with people of several populations in various settings, including hospitals and community mental health.

Katie DiCola graduated from Mercy College in August 2020 with a Masters of Science in Psychology. She is currently working in the field as an educational liaison within the Pediatric Division of Hematology, Oncology, & Stem Cell Transplantation at Columbia University Medical Center. Her research interests include health psychology, pediatric oncology and school psychology.

Joanna N. Dovalis MA PhD is a marriage and family therapist with a doctorate in clinical psychology, specializing in grief work. She has authored several chapters in books on Jung and film published by Routledge. Recently, she coauthored a book with John Izod titled, *Cinema as Therapy: Grief in Transformational Film*, which was recently published by Routledge. She works in private practice in southern California, USA.

Dr. Gaetano Giordano, MD, has a medical sciences and surgery degree with a specialty in psychotherapy and forensic medicine. He is president of the Analytical Psychology Institute and a professor at Chieti University. Dr. Giordano was an early adopter of using the creative aspects of videotape as part of his therapeutic practice and is a consultant in filmsettings and television programs. He also works in Rome, Italy, as a forensic scientist and psychotherapist, with a focus on separation and divorce.

Christopher R. Harz, EdD, MBA, has worked extensively in virtual reality (VR) worlds and simulations, as an analyst at the RAND Corporation and for DoD and the Intelligence Community. He was a producer of the $240 million SIMNET (the first massively multiplayer online game) project for DARPA and NATOnet for NATO allies, among others. Dr. Harz is working on game development and use for therapy and performance improvement for the DoD. His doctoral thesis examined the role of end-user involvement in videogame development. He has a doctorate in Educational Technology from Pepperdine University, and MBA and BA (Psychology) degrees.

Nancy Mramor Kajuth, PhD, founded Transformedia, LLC, to create transformational media for personal growth. The types of media include television, radio, articles, books, and blogs, as well as workshops, lectures, and individual sessions for therapy and coaching. Both of her major book releases have received author awards in the categories of self-help and the bridge between spirituality and consciousness. In her spare time, she has taught on the adjunct faculty of five Pennsylvania Universities and participates in the American Psychological Association Media Division. Her creation and research of a multimedia curriculum for children entitled Mastering Relaxation, proved to be highly effective in reducing symptoms of stress.

Yarden Kerem, MA, has a master of fine arts (MFA) degree and is based in Jerusalem, Israel. A practicing psychotherapist focusing on ways that pay attention to the somatic experience, with specialization on attachment and trauma. Member of the European Association of Body Psychotherapy (EARP).

An authorized coordinator ordained by the International Institute of Focusing. Supervisor of therapists dealing with physical focusing

using the reference or attitude treatment. She established the Focusing School of photo and video therapy and the Center for Therapy through Video in the Ma'ale Film School in Jerusalem. She has developed and written study courses on therapy through video. She produced and directed documentary films. She holds an M.FA from Tel Aviv University in fine arts and an MA in therapy through expression and creativity. She also holds a BA in philosophy from the Hebrew University of Jerusalem, and was a contributor to the book *Video, and Filmmaking as Psychotherapy: Research and Practice* (Cohen, Johnson, & Orr, 2015), published by Routledge.

Kimberly Marynowski graduated from Florida State University with a BS in Psychology and earned her MA in Psychology from Hunter College, where she created a novel paradigm under Dr. Dennis-Tiwary, successfully manipulating phubbing in face-to-face interaction in a controlled lab setting. She is currently a doctoral student in the Clinical Psychology Ph.D. program at Palo Alto University and a Student Therapist at the Gronowski Clinic. Her research interests include health psychology, integrated health, digital interventions and mindfulness meditation.

Penelope P. Orr, PhD, ATR-BC, is a board-certified registered art therapist. She is an Art Therapy Board credentialed supervisor; has served on the Art Therapy Credentials Board, which credentials all art therapists in the United States; and was the president of this board from January 2011 to December 2013. She has taught at Edinboro University and Florida State University for the past ten years, over which time she published one book, wrote chapters for two edited books, and published 15 articles on digital media theory and use in art therapy. She is a contributor to the book *Video and Filmmaking as Psychotherapy: Research and Practice* (Cohen, Johnson, & Orr, 2015), published by Routledge.

Lila Pereira, PhD, is Narrative and Trauma in Cancer research Assistant Professor of Pediatrics and Psychiatry at New York Medical College Valhalla, New York, and Summary Licensed Psychologist in New York State. Following are her specialty areas and research focus: Pediatric Psychology, Psycho-oncology, Adjustment to Chronic Illness, Chronic Illness Transition to Adulthood (AYA), Integrated Healthcare, Social Media as a Support Tool, Video Illness Narratives, AYA, and LGBTQ Health. She recently coauthored a peer-reviewed article titled "Factors Related to Linguistic Content in Video Narrative of Adolescents with Cancer and Healthy Controls."

Rodríguez Pérez, R. N., PhD, is a Video Art Therapist and Gestalt Therapist. She is an Honorary Professor at the Autónoma University in Madrid, Spain. She holds a PhD in Fine Arts from Politécnica University in Valencia, Spain. She also holds a master's degree in Visual and Multimedia Arts from the UPV, and a master's degree in Art Therapy from UVIC and AEC in Barcelona, Spain.

Her current projects include pursuing a degree in Psychology and developing the educational, recreational, therapeutic, and creative project "La Escuela de lo que no sabemos" (The School of the Undiscovered), of which she is the cofounder.

Dr. Albert "Skip" Rizzo, PhD, is a clinical psychologist and Director of Medical Virtual Reality at the University of Southern California Institute for Creative Technologies. He is also a research professor with the USC Department of Psychiatry and at the USC Davis School of Gerontology. Over the last 20 years, Rizzo has conducted research on the design, development, and evaluation of Virtual Reality systems targeting the areas of clinical assessment,and rehabilitation across the domains of psychological, cognitive, and motor functioning in both healthy and clinical populations. This work has focused on PTSD, TBI, Autism, ADHD, Alzheimer's disease, stroke, and other clinical conditions. In spite of the diversity of these clinical R&D areas, the common thread that drives all of his work with digital technologies involves the study of how interactive and immersive Virtual Reality simulations can be usefully applied to address human healthcare needs beyond what is possible with traditional twentieth-century tools and methods. To view some videos of this work, please visit this YouTube channel: http://www.youtube.com/user/albertskiprizzo.

Bronwyn Robertson, LPC, MSED, is a licensed professional counselor who has lectured and published internationally on integrative psychotherapy for trauma and anxiety. She has more than 25 years' experience working with individuals with trauma-related disorders in community-based, outpatient, inpatient, and residential settings. She works with all age groups and specializes in working with individuals who have complex trauma histories including children in foster care and individuals with developmental disabilities. She specializes in mindfulness-based psychotherapy for anxiety, stress, panic, trauma, depression, and mood disorders. Her training and certifications include EMDR Level 1, trauma model therapy, acceptance and commitment therapy, mindfulness-based CBT, trauma-focused CBT, and somatic experiencing. She integrates mindfulness-based cinematherapy and trauma-focused cognitive-behavioral therapy with somatic experiencing, expressive and play therapy approaches in individual, group, and family therapy. She has a private practice and works with nonprofit agencies in Virginia.

Myriam D. Savage PhD, RDT-BCT, is a registered drama therapist and Southern California and chapter president of the North American Drama Therapy Association. She is a faculty lecturer at the UCLA School of Arts and Architecture: Visual Arts and Performing arts program for Greater Los Angeles. She worked for the UCLArts and Healing program, called Social Emotional Arts (SEA), which teaches art educators, therapists, and artists holistic ways of working with various populations using the arts.

Sascha Schneider holds a master of forensic science (MFS) degree from the Phillips Institute. He was one of the cofounders of the Second Generation group in Los Angeles. He has been one of the facilitators for the German-Jewish dialogue groups for "One by One" in Berlin, dialogue between children of Holocaust survivors and children of Nazis. Sascha has been in the film industry since 1966 and has worked on numerous documentaries from David Wolper Productions, as well as many TV series, including *Hill Street Blues*.

Sascha and Lauren Schneider are the producers-directors of the award-winning documentary *Chuppa*, which deals with the family affect and resolution of a Holocaust survivor family.

Alina Skrzeszewska, MA, is an award-winning documentary filmmaker. She was born in Poland, raised in Germany, and currently is based in Los Angeles. She holds a diploma in stage design and experimental media from the University of the Arts Berlin, as well as an MFA in Film and Video from the California Institute of the Arts. Alina has spent close to a decade exploring the complex neighborhood of L.A.'s infamous Skid Row in various film projects, among them the award-winning feature documentary *Songs from the Nickel* and, most recently, *Game Girls*.

Dr. Valentina Stoycheva received her doctoral degree in Clinical Psychology from the Derner Institute for Advanced Psychological Studies at Adelphi University, Garden City, NY. She completed her predoctoral internship at Kings County Hospital in Brooklyn and a postdoctoral fellowship specializing in military and trauma psychology at the Unified Behavioral Health Center for Military Personnel and their Families, Northwell Health. She has received specialized trainings in utilizing empirically based treatments (EBTs) for PTSD, depression, and anxiety disorders, as well as couples/family psychotherapy, and Trauma-Focused Cognitive Behavioral Treatment (TF-CBT) for children. Dr. Stoycheva has worked extensively within the field of trauma—ranging from early childhood abuse to domestic violence, to surviving natural disasters and war-related trauma—as well as with anxiety and panic disorders, mood disorders, and personality disorders. She is a Certified Clinical Trauma Professional. The scope of her experience includes working with children, adolescents, adults, and families, in both inpatient and outpatient settings. Her approach is integrative, blending psychodynamic, relational, cognitive-behavioral, and dialectical-behavioral techniques, tailored individually for each client. Dr. Stoycheva has also held a two-year Research Fellowship at the Pacella Parent-Child Center, New York Psychoanalytic Institute. She has taught both undergraduate- and graduate-level college courses and has contributed over a dozen publications and presentations in the fields of trauma, family dynamics, and the psychotherapy process. Dr. Stoycheva is a member of the American Psychological Association (APA), of Division 56 (Trauma Division) of APA, of the International Society for Traumatic Stress Studies (ISTSS), and of the Suffolk County Psychological Association. She is a coauthor of *The Unconscious: Theory, Research, and Clinical Implications*— winner of the 2021 Book Prize in Theory of the American Board and Academy of Psychoanalysis. The book focuses on how everyday unconscious processes shape our beliefs, attitudes, thoughts, behaviors, and the psychotherapy process. You can also read Dr. Stoycheva's article series The Everyday Unconscious on *Psychology Today*.

Foreword

Albert "Skip" Rizzo

The experience of trauma is ubiquitous and comes in many forms. Trauma also knows no boundaries across the lifespan. Children exposed to adverse childhood experiences involving abuse, neglect, and household dysfunction often sustain long-term negative impacts on their physical and mental health (Bhushan et al., 2020). Senior citizens routinely suffer from loss and traumatic grief, whether due to the death of a lifelong significant other or to the gradual or unexpected loss of function, or with the fear and anxiety that accompanies the sudden awareness of having a life-ending disease process. And at every point in between, there is no shortage of human exposure to a wide variety of traumatic life experiences due to physical/emotional/sexual assault, motor vehicle and other forms of injury/accidents, wartime exposure, extreme weather, becoming a refugee, marital breakups, and debilitating disease processes. Regardless of one's clinical orientation, most care providers consensually agree that successful coping with such adversity is not naturally endowed or consistently applied in many people who go on to suffer chronic and enduring negative reactions to traumatic experiences. When viewed in this wider context, it would not be a stretch to say that clinical care practitioners and researchers spend much of their careers primarily focused on the reduction of human pain and suffering due to exposure to traumatic life events.

Throughout human history, many healthcare practices have been evolved that aim to reduce or manage trauma-based suffering via pharmacological agents, talk therapies, exercise, and spiritual practices, among many thousands of other approaches. Despite the existence of these treatment approaches, trauma survivors are often unaware of them, or due to a negative bias inherent in the response to traumatic stress, many trauma-exposed sufferers do not believe that they will achieve benefit from the effort that may be involved in any therapeutic activity. This subset of barriers to care results in a population of "walking wounded" B human beings who might otherwise be helped if they engaged with treatment (Rizzo & Koenig, 2017). The relevance of efforts to break down such barriers to mental health care can be starkly seen in the World

Health Organization (WHO) estimate that over 450 million people suffer with a known mental health condition, of which fully two-thirds will never see the inside of a therapy office (2001, 2018)! The WHO also predicts that by the year 2030 mental health conditions will be the leading burden of disease globally (2021). Thus, clinical strategies need to evolve and take a form that not only is supported by scientific evidence but also serves to reduce barriers to care by their appealing nature and wide availability.

One potential remedy for this global challenge may be derived from the recent advances in information and computing technology that have birthed a new class of general mental health treatment strategies that could have significant impact on traumatic stress care (Cukor et al., 2009; Rizzo et al., 2021). This involves the emergence of new media technology (internet-based therapy, mobile applications, virtual/augmented reality, etc.), in addition to a reexamination of the power of more traditional forms of media, particularly cinema.

Certainly, there is a long history of media having a pervasive impact on the advancement of humanity and civilization. The diverse forms and mechanisms of such media is breathtaking—from cave paintings, sometimes with faux animation effects delivered via the flickering light of a campfire (Azéma & Rivère, 2012), to early forms of written text, sculpting, and painting, to the output of Gutenberg's fifteenth-century printing press, to the first zoetrope in 1833, through to the growth and availability of radio, cinema, television, and even graphic novels (comic books) across the twentieth century. There can be no doubt that media representations have served to give many people a window into the imaginations, events, and "virtual" worlds conceived by others, that would otherwise be unseen. This power to create and represent life experiences for the consumption of others has been exponentially amplified with the advent of mass deliverable and interactive media content that computing and internet technologies have enabled since the 1990s. Those who choose to ignore the potential to leverage these technological advances to support the delivery of mental health and wellness strategies do so at their own (or their patients') peril.

All media forms share a common ability to entertain, document, educate, and inform, and now we must add to this list, the capacity to heal! Certainly, media has always had some role in promoting health. Health concepts have a long history of appearing in media, whether appearing in a cave painting to characterize danger or to promote survival during the hunt, or, for better or worse, cautionary tales about the impact and existential consequences of bad "character" (or lack of religious faith) have been staples in narrative print, audio, stage acting, and "moving pictures." Such narrative often includes common prescriptions and exhortations for leading a "good" life that, from the author's perspective, deserved to be modeled. Now, with the advent of more widely distributed, connected, and interactive media, the potential for positive (and negative) mental health impact has only grown! Thus, the potency for using both traditional and new media as a positive driver and influence on mental health demands a deep analysis to support more thoughtful and comprehensive investigations as to the benefits that could be accrued, as well as the risks, from a fully connected global "metaverse." This is what is so compelling about *Film/Video-Based Therapy™ and Trauma: Research and Practice*. In one package, this fascinating book presents expert perspectives on the power of film, video games, mixed reality, etc., to create new strategies for dealing with the impact of trauma, as well as for improving mental health more generally.

One of the key elements discussed in this book, and one of the more potent components of these technology-based approaches, is in their capacity to educate and inform via the strategic use of storytelling. In addition to the known value of direct experiential learning, following the narrative of another's experience in facing and coping with life challenges is a powerful method for learning and self-understanding. Leveraging the power of narrative can provide the building blocks for helping a person to construct a road map for individual change that supports a path toward improved mental health. When these processes are activated by engagement with cinema and other new media formats, the potential for improving mental health and well-being becomes obvious. These media options allow individuals to observe and emotionally engage with the impact of adversity on others and promote self-reflection as to how the viewer might approach a similar challenge in their own life. Such experiences, albeit through passive observation, have been evolved in the genetics of humanity as scientists have documented the capacity of mirror neurons in the brain to build mental templates for implementing real action in the world. Now imagine the additive impact of advanced immersive narrative VR worlds that go beyond passive observation by endowing the user with the capacity to make choices that effect the direction of the story in real time. This format would then allow a person to test out an infinite number of "What if" scenarios, but in a safe context where the outcomes of user choice can inform rather than harm.

Cinematic portrayals in both traditional and new media can also play a strong role in increasing empathy for the suffering of others! Certainly, tragic stagecraft and cinema have a long history in this area, but new media technologies like virtual reality can deliver emotionally evocative, first-person empathy experiences, the power of which researchers have now begun to document. These interactive experiences within simulated worlds serve to drive both experiential learning and the power of narrative to activate the user's imagination for considering the varied opportunities for coping and empathy-building that are rarely available in real-life interactions without significant risk or cost.

Thus, the nature and content of this book should excite anyone with an interest in improving the mental health status of the world at a time when the challenges of scorched-earth political conflict, economic/racial inequality, environmental threats, the questioning of the value of expertise, and a global pandemic have whipped the masses into a state of stressful apprehension, dystopian anxiety, and alternating bouts of abject desperation and apathy. If there was ever a time when mental health scientists and media artists needed to come together to address the mental health ills of the human condition, it is now. Whereas, for better or worse, the Industrial Age in Western society served to reduce much of the physical suffering that humans have faced over thousands of years of survival, let us hope that the bounty of the Information Age will likewise reduce some of the mental suffering. This book arrives at a moment when thoughtful consideration and exploration of the impact of media-driven narrative and experiential learning is not just timely, but necessary.

References

Azéma, M., & Rivère, F. (2012). Animation in Palaeolithic art: A pre-echo of cinema. *Antiquity*, 86(332), 316–324.

Bhushan, D., Kotz, K., McCall, J., Wirtz, S., Gilgoff, R., Dube, S. R., Powers, C., Olson-Morgan, J., Galeste, M., Patterson, K., Harris, L., Mills, A., Bethell, C., & Burke-Harris, N. (2020). *Roadmap for resilience: The California Surgeon General's report on adverse childhood experiences, toxic stress, and health.* Office of the California Surgeon General. doi: 10.48019/PEAM8812

Cukor, J., Spitalnick, J., Difede, J., Rizzo, A., & Rothbaum, B. O. (2009). Emerging treatments for PTSD. *Clinical Psychology Review*, 29(8), 715–726.

Rizzo, A., Hartholt, A., & Mozgai, S. (2021). Establishment of clinical virtual reality methodologies from the front lines of Afghanistan to COVID-19. In: W. Greenleaf, L. Roberts, & R. Fine (Eds.), *Applied virtual reality in healthcare: Case studies and perspectives* (pp. 163–188). Cool Blue Media.

Rizzo, A., & Koenig, S. (2017). Is clinical virtual reality ready for primetime? *Neuropsychology*, 31(8). doi: 10.1037/neu0000405

World Health Organization. (2001). *The World Health Report 2001: Mental health: New understanding, new hope.* Author.

World Health Organization. (2018). *Mental health atlas 2017.* Author.

World Health Organization. (2021). *Comprehensive mental health action plan 2013–2030.* https://apps.who.int/iris/bitstream/handle/10665/345301/9789240031029-eng.pdf?sequence=1

Acknowledgments

This book is intended to inspire posttraumatic growth.

I want to thank many people who helped make this book happen. First, David Israelian and Peer Mental Health for their financial support. Diane Johns for her tireless work in the formatting and APA style. The many authors and people involved in the military and the American Psychological Association for their support and the international support for the book, including people from the Czech Republic, Netherlands, Brazil, Australia, Italy, Romania, Spain, Israel, Egypt, Canada, England, and more mentioned in www.filmandvideobasedtherapy.com.

Like the first book, *Video and Filmmaking as Psychotherapy: Research and Practice*, the idea for this book began in 1997. The seminar on Cinematherapy ™ I hosted at Colorado College introduced the concept to an undergraduate population. Since then, I've discovered how many various people have contributed to film/video-based therapy independently over the years since the 1940s in group homes. Many of them recently were art therapists.

I want to thank Dr. Albert "Skip" Rizzo for his involvement in the Peer Mental Health (PMH) mixer, the foreword to the book, and my presentation to Sharon Israel's school in Israel on virtual reality and filmmaking. With the invention of Virtual Reality, the possibility of making films is even more viable with virtual film sets.

I also want to thank the authors who presented at the PMH mixer in Los Angeles and beyond in both the University of Southern California, especially Lynn Crandall at the USC IGM Art Gallery, for her moral support and ability to bring the country together as a former award recipient from the Barack Obama White House.

There is a second volume in process with many authors who are not entirely in this version and who are mentioned in the introduction and later on the website as well, including Elyn Saks, a distinguished mental health law professor at the University of Southern California, who was interviewed for the second volume of this book and discussed how stigma and ethics might apply to Film/Video-Based Therapy and Virtual Reality.

Peer Mental Health and AnaVault, a psychological corporation, were helpful to the book because they put ideas into practice The second book will also go into more detail about the current or potential future research including work with neuroTree (https://www.neurotree.io/ also found in www.filmandvideobasedtherapy.com). This book focuses explicitly on trauma and while not about one theorist or the other, focuses on triggers and the process of healing. lso, I owea debt to both Peter Levine and Bessel van der Kolk's ideas. I trained under Peter Levine's Somatic Experiencing program for up to three years. There is a long, unofficial backstory to this book which is noted in private through a series of hour-long films through Your Digital Storytelling Project, Peer Mental Health, and the University of Southern California, which serves in place of an experimental film in response to the pandemic and which demonstrates that this process works.

I hope this book will foster future research in trauma like it did when Benjamin Patton and Rivka Tuval-Mashiach published with Charles Drebbing in a later clinical trial.

Trauma is not about the event; however, after COVID this topic is especially relevant. The bleak reality of death and suffering resulting in job loss, PTSD, depression, and cognitive decline due to COVID are untracked entirely, and we do not know the long-term effects of the pandemic's psychological and economic impact. I would also like to acknowledge the brave men and women who helped fight COVID in hospital settings and found the strength to face this overwhelming loss. I had COVID and pneumonia while on dialysis before the vaccine and saw many colleagues and friends die, as others have. There is no chapter about COVID in this book because it was written before the onset of COVID. In addition, this book is about the process of coping with trauma, not the incidents or triggers specifically. To see my response to COVID, please visit my professional work. at www.yourdigitalstorytellingproject.com. Trauma theorists can be said to believe that trauma is not about one's personal narrative but rather more, as Peter Levine says in his work, about a response to overwhelming experiences that shut down one's normal flow of functioning.

I'm deeply grateful to the authors who contributed to this volume, and despite their struggles over the years, they remained able to finish their part in this work.

Although I wish I could have spent more time with family and friends in person, I'm grateful for their virtual presence and support during the pandemic and the production of the book. Although the book was created during physical isolation, one can sense the felt presence of their support everywhere.

Thank you all for supporting me in integrating the darkness and light into my life through story.

Part I
Introduction

1 Film/Video-Based Therapy™ and Virtual Reality

Joshua L. Cohen

> So in the Avengers, as in the other Marvel groups, it is the collective forces, rather than the ego-driven solo hero, that provides the redeeming energy for humankind.
>
> —Anslow (2012, p. 242)

This book uses film/video-based therapy™ to help build resilience in facing personal, communal, national, and global trauma triggers. Reducing trauma can be a challenge in any circumstance and may involve collaboration. Filmmaking is a collaborative process, and similar to the movie, *The Avengers*, no single person can address global trauma alone. This is an edited book that focuses on collaboration in addressing trauma. We address issues in one's home, community, country, and the world using integrative medicine and advocacy using film/video-based therapy™ and digital storytelling to address trauma in one's home, community, government, and the world. This book is designed to be used by the audience of practitioners in the field and educators in higher education institutions. The previous book, *Video and Filmmaking as Psychotherapy: Research and Practice* (Cohen, Johnson, & Orr, 2015), introduced film/video-based therapy™ as a new approach to psychotherapy and explored various theoretical backgrounds and approaches as well as ethical dilemmas that might be inherent to its practice in an interdisciplinary way of thinking contrary to more independent thought. The concept of synergy and focus is not unfamiliar to the filmmaker who works with many different art forms (Cohen, 2022). This second book expands on the topic of the first book; it is about how therapy using film and video can heal both individuals and communities by helping people find their place in a community for both purpose and life energy that motivates and inspires despite the traumatic events one might face.

The world has suffered—and continues to suffer—collective trauma, terrorism, and violence. As a result, mental health professionals, creative art therapists, filmmakers, and activists working as researchers and practitioners are faced with daunting challenges. This book demonstrates how we can use the language of film to watch, process, and discuss images

DOI: 10.4324/9781315622507-2

of trauma in therapy, in the home, in the community, and in the world (Cohen et al., 2015).

Psychological Trauma

Trauma is not just about the experience, not only at the time of the event. It is about one's subsequent response to triggers, as described by pioneer trauma researchers and practitioners such as Bessel van der Kolk, Peter Levine, and other depth psychologists, and in qualitative and quantitative research. In this book on the topic of digital storytelling as therapy (Film/Video-Based Therapy™) (Cohen, 2022), we build on the work of the first book, *Video and Filmmaking as Psychotherapy: Research and Practice* (Cohen et al., 2015), which examined film/video-based theory across issues and populations in a general sense.

This book demonstrates those theories in a new way by focusing on posttraumatic growth through media psychology, depth psychology, neuroscience, medicine, and advocacy's role in using film/video-based therapy™. A psychotherapy client needs to have become aware of all triggers of trauma to help build resilience in the face of overwhelming experiences for the sake of regulating the autonomic nervous system (Cohen et al., 2015).

Film/video-based therapy™ can help a client not only to become aware of those triggers and learn how they can be processed personally but also to become an advocate for change using digital storytelling and by learning how to process triggers in the home, local community, state, country, and the world that may otherwise leave one vulnerable to trauma.

Definition of Film/Video-Based Therapy™

Film/Video-Based Therapy™ involves making movies with clients. It also draws from several disciplines, including cinema therapy, expressive therapy, narrative therapy, art therapy, digital storytelling, and phototherapy. The making of any film involves a community that requires collaboration to integrate the many dynamic aspects of art and medicine. A collaborative effort was formed around film/video-based therapy™ to demonstrate health in community settings. Film/Video-Based Therapy™ is about *making* films with clients, in contrast to cinema therapy ™, which involves *watching* films. I have utilized watching movies and mindfulness in my work. I have also been cited in Tuval-Mashiach and Patton's clinical trial and participated in peer-reviewed research on the use of video narratives in cancer research. Film/Video-Based Therapy™ is not trademarked for advertising or financial purposes; rather, it is intended to protect the sanctity of the license for mental health professionals and the word "therapy" when used in conjunction with film/video in the United States (Cohen et al., 2015).

Somatic Experiencing and Trauma

Somatic Experiencing, in its simplest terms, is more of a mind-body practice than a psychological practice. Somatic Experiencing practitioner Paul Petschek demonstrated this in an interview in which I allowed him to draw from his cinematic experience editing with directors like Martin Scorsese and Thelma Schoonmaker to explain whether Levine's idea of SIBAM would work perfectly with film editing. (SIBAM stands for Sensation, Image, Behavior, Affect, and Meaning and will be expanded on throughout the book.)

> SE is a body-oriented therapeutic model applied in multiple professions and professional settings—psychotherapy, medicine, coaching, teaching, and physical therapy. Trauma impacts physical health, mental health, learning, education, and multiple aspects of an individual's life.
>
> (About—Somatic Experiencing® International [2021, November 9])

Bessel Van Der Kolk and Trauma: *The Body Keeps the Score*

Bessel van der Kolk's work, *The Body Keeps the Score*, was on the number one list of the *New York Times*'s bestsellers. He is one of the world's leading experts on traumatic stress. In his book, he explains how psychological trauma influences people as well as how to move beyond it (van der Kolk, 2015).

Dr. Albert "Skip" Rizzo: Exposure Therapy and VR

In his interview with Brett Leonard about the movie *Lawnmower Man*, Skip Rizzo explored how VR looked in the future from a 1990s perspective. New films like *The Matrix* series use the Unreal Engine, not for virtual reality, but the gaming engine. It helps provide for cinematic form in movies (Rizzo, 2021; Wachowski, 2022).

Psychologist Skip Rizzo researches the design, development, and evaluation of virtual reality (VR) systems targeting the areas of clinical assessment, treatment rehabilitation, and resilience. This work spans psychological, cognitive, and motor functioning domains in both healthy and clinical populations. Rizzo, whose work uses virtual reality-based exposure therapy to treat PTSD, holds research professor appointments with the USC Department of Psychiatry and Behavioral Sciences and the USC Davis School of Gerontology (Cognitive Technology; Journal of Computer Animation and Virtual Worlds; Media Psychology) and is the creator of the Virtual Reality Mental Health Email Listserv (VRPSYCH).

The Mandalorian, Virtual Filmmaking, and the Unreal Engine

The unreal engine and Disney and Lucasfilm have designed a gaming engine perfect for film/video-based therapy™ and Patton's "I Was There" Films workshops (Cohen et al., 2015; Rizzo, 2021).

Disney's incredible series *The Mandalorian* used the Unreal Engine for sets (L.A. Castle Studios, 2020). We are also working with Unreal Engine with authors in Canada and Egypt for the second volume of *Film/Video-Based Therapy™ and Trauma*. The Mandalorian used Unreal for most of the reasons that help with constricting costs and the ability to mix physical props with virtual sets (Gartenberg, 2020). It helps in therapy because of HIPAA and other restrictions for filmmaking in the therapy room.

Film/Video-Based Therapy™, Trauma Backstory, and Chapter Summaries

When I started working on this book, it was 2016, and I was looking at trauma through the lens of psychological problems. At that time, people had survived 9/11, the war in Iraq, and the United States's extended conflict in Afghanistan. All the traumas at that time had to do with terrorism and the military. We didn't expect a medical crisis. The global coronavirus pandemic forced us to confront the medical issues in our communities as people focused on the health of their families while relatives, friends, and strangers died slowly, and the world shut down. But nothing could prepare us for what happened to mental health in the aftermath of the pandemic. From a mental health perspective, trying to jump-start a system that was already broken was horrifying, challenging, and almost impossible.

While it is a continuation of *Video and Filmmaking as Psychotherapy: Research and Practice*, this book is centered on the concept of psychological trauma. I chose this topic because of the possibility for inspiration it can foster when associated with posttraumatic growth. Unlike physical trauma, psychological trauma has particular qualities. Whereas physical trauma is about the incident, psychological trauma is unique to the response. Psychological trauma is less about what happened and more about one's reaction to that trigger. Hence, it leaves room for posttraumatic growth. If you have psychological trauma, you can neither fight nor retreat from a situation. To use an automotive analogy, it's like simultaneously flooring the gas pedal and slamming on the brakes.

For years I studied Peter Levine's methods, taking his classes on Somatic Experiencing, but became ill before I could obtain the final credential. COVID-19 interfered with much of the progress I had made. Levine's work coincided with that of Bessel van der Kolk, who published a *New York Times* bestselling paperback titled *The Body Keeps the Score: Brain, Mind, and Body in the Healing of Trauma* (2015). Levine (1997) and van der Kolk had collaborated before and supported each other's work in the past. Although different in method and theory, each upholds the tenet that trauma resides in the body and requires techniques designed to stabilize a person who has undergone a horrendous, life-changing experience.

This book, while it is about technology, is focused on using technology to better explain—in my interpretation through the author's lens—the concept of the body, its role in processing trauma, and how we deal with trauma to make things better. I originally intended the book's subtitle to include the words "post-traumatic growth." As you explore the different chapters, you'll see that they all overtly or covertly incorporate Peter Levine's principle of somatic experiencing as well as those of similar theorists.

From a global perspective, the concept of how trauma can have a ripple effect on the world starts with the individual. An individual can influence a person's family, and they can influence their community. That community can influence the city, which will affect the state, the country, and eventually the world. This is how the book is organized, based on Natalie Rogers's concept of person-centered peace (Rogers, 2012).

The concept is inherently bipartisan because all mammals have a nervous system. The parasympathetic and sympathetic parts of the autonomic nervous system focus on Somatic Experiencing and, to some degree, all trauma work. In this book, we will be using storytelling through Film/Video-Based Therapy™ and virtual reality to regulate people suffering from trauma and to have a ripple effect on the world.

This researcher believes that all parts of the *Diagnostic and Statistical Manual* have to do with dysregulation of the autonomic nervous system. Throughout the book, we will learn more about the influence of both Levine and van der Kolk and their influence on this field through other theorists who have worked with them.

Part II: Trauma in the Home, City, State/Province

Dr. Valentina Stoycheva explores how trauma work brings up the use of metaphors. She provides background on biological work like that of Stephen Porges and the polyvagal theory. She ties the theme of trauma Film/Video-Based Therapy™ via storytelling and the veteran population. She also presents a couple of cases as examples of how her metaphors and trauma connect with certain veterans as she works with that population.

Bronwyn Robertson writes about a relatively new concept called neurocinematics. She draws from integrated practices like neuroscience, brain imaging, and the body. This chapter explores how neurocinematics, a specific branch of neuroscience, can be effectively and ethically applied within trauma therapy. Robertson highlights cases in which neurocinematics were applied within integrative trauma therapies, mindfulness-based and Somatic Experiencing (SE) practices.

Dr. Chris Harz uses virtual reality to discuss how VR games can produce a healthy environment for dealing with various conditions, including posttraumatic stress disorder. Chris has worked with the military on research, including the RAND Corporation. He notes,

A number of videogames exist for phobias such as fear of flying or claustrophobia, involving the use of VR for exposure therapy .... However, experience has shown that one-size-fits-all game worlds may not be optimal, and that user input and some customization of the virtual sets could make the therapy more immersive .... Addictions to drugs, gambling, and other repetitive stimulants tend to involve a failure to recognize patterns and denial of the likely consequences of a behavior pattern.

In the next chapter, Dr. Penelope P. Orr returns as an author for the second book in a row. She talks about her research as a Fulbright scholar and turns the lens on herself as she goes through a challenging breast cancer journey. It *was* a challenge; I imagine that it was grueling to write this chapter. Once you read it, you'll have the opportunity to understand what a fantastic accomplishment it is by spending some time learning about her journey.

Part III: Trauma in the United States

Dr. Leila Pereira and her co-authors focus on how storytelling through video is used with adolescent and young adult (AYA) cancer patients, who make video testimonials similar to those seen on YouTube as a way to process their cancer experience. The video stories and testimonials are similar to Carolyn McGurl et al.'s work in *Video and Filmmaking Psychotherapy: Research and Practice*.

Dr. Joanna Dovalis analyzes *The Wolfpack*, a documentary about children confined by their father in a New York City apartment who use filmmaking to stay alive. Joanna has been published in Europe, and she works with a collection of post-Jungian thinkers who use film to express and explain their approach to Jungian psychotherapy. She holds a Ph.D. in Clinical Psychology from Pacifica Graduate Institute and has practiced under her MFT license for many years.

Nancy Mramor Kajuth's chapter focuses on many different aspects of film and production. In her examination of Pete Docter's *Inside Out*, she looks at emotions. She also introduces other films, including *The Upside of Anger*, about which she says,

As a psychologist and producer for PBS-TV, creating a window into the world and the mind for viewers was a rewarding task. The production of psychology segments for an evening news show brought the elements of understanding the self and how we become who we are to the screen.

Part IV: Trauma in the World

The next chapter is a story told by Sascha Schneider about how his parents never got married after they survived the Holocaust. Schneider is a film and television producer who produced shows in the 1980s, including *Hill Street Blues* and many films. In this case, he turned the camera on his own family. His documentary, *Chuppah (The Wedding Canopy)*, won several awards for the inspiring way he portrayed how his mother and father married 50 years after surviving the Holocaust. The film depicts his family and their survival in overcoming German oppression during the Holocaust.

Dr. Gaetano Giordano talks about video movie therapy in Italy. He gives a history of Italian cinema, including Italian comedies, up to the current age. In his practice, Giordano uses video technology to tell the story of the group and client. He does so as a clinician in the service of the client, not the audience. Ethically, this approach does not violate patient confidentiality. He strictly recommends that all video movie therapy participants also stay involved in individual therapy. What makes his process work is the enjoyment aspect.

In the next chapter, we turn to Nerea Rodriguez Pérez's work, which considers an art therapy and video approach to Gestalt therapy, psychoanalysis, and holism. She looks at it as the driving force of the process: this has been confirmed in the description and analysis of practice. It is essential to pay attention to the position from which each participant viewed the process and address what they chose to focus on. It took into account the gaze of both the patient and the video art therapist, and the view each took of the production. Dr. Pérez and her work in Spain allowed her to get a different perspective. In her country, as they developed video therapy in universities and her particular form and take on it, they also enacted other laws and regulations ethically, which give a different perspective.

The next chapter reviews the award-winning film and group support project titled *Game Girls* that combined documentary filmmaking with drama/expressive therapy. It helped shed light on the narratives of homeless women on Skid Row, Los Angeles, over a two-year period. The documentary witnessed the transformation of the lives of two women in their environment. The production team also grew from the documented stories. Within the film, they formed friendships and bonded with people in the community that helped shaped their challenges as well as fostered healing. Years after the release of the film, the filmmaker, drama therapist, and various people in the community of that film witnessed both trauma and growth and looking back saw also healing that grew from the relationships built. Within most films, it is the therapeutic relationship that was likely the source of healing and the film created the space for that healing to take place.

Brooke Campbell writes about drama therapy. In her chapter, she discusses the aesthetics of theatre and how it relates to trauma. To support her theory, she also describes an interview with Robert Landy. Landy is famous in his field for his work with drama therapy and some of the positive educational outcomes of working with the theater and clinical practices and evidence-based outcomes.

Introduction to Volume 2

This book had to be broken into two parts to accommodate the number of authors and topics after COVID-19. Considering it's about global trauma, we did a good job condensing the material. First, we will discuss ethics with Elyn Saks and Alex Elliott.

Elyn Saks is a mental health advocate, scholar, and recipient of the MacArthur Genius Award. She spoke about how her success in incorporating her diagnosis of schizophrenia as a mental health law professor at USC has helped transform the system and prepared other people to deal with mental health from a legal point of view. Her TED talk about her story and her list of publications can be found here: https://filmandvideobasedtherapy.com/

I met Elyn through David Israelian and Barbara Wilson at the Saks Institute at USC filmandvideobasedtherapy.com. We discussed psychiatric medication and the stigma of mental illness in the recorded interview clips from that interview. She let me know what her students were saying about stigma and how it could affect getting help.

Incidentally, my Ph.D. dissertation also applies to mental health stigma, as it addressed the space to allow one's identity to transform through the identification of being an artist (filmandvideobasedtherapy.com). Making art allows the freedom to transform an individual's identity. When doing a project, the patient takes on a new identity, which keeps them from identifying as someone with a mental health challenge and makes them think of themselves as more artist than patient.

Alex Elliott is a psychiatric social worker who works in Los Angeles County. Alex and I also met through David Israelian. We talked about the county programs in the recorded interview (http://filmandvideobasedtherapy.com/). Alex Elliott also talked about his struggle with physical disabilities. He used virtual reality for his disability and demonstrated it at a recorded public event for Peer Mental Health. He also showed how it could be incorporated into his work as a psychiatric social worker in Los Angeles County. Alex and I also discussed many other issues in the interview recorded in 2020 that apply to stigma and mental health law and ethics.

Dr. Albert "Skip" Rizzo, the designated author of Volume 1's foreword, is one of the leading medical directors of the Institute of Creative Technologies at the University of Southern California (Rizzo, 2022). His work with virtual reality and project Bravemind has allowed them to help us narrow the gap between virtual reality and the film industry. After working with Benjamin Patton's company (described in the previous book), they later developed a clinical trial that cited my work (http://filmandvideobasedtherapy.com/). Dr. Rizzo also works with trauma in the military and other programs with patients suffering from many different conditions, including ADHD, autism, and cerebral palsy. He presented those interventions in collaboration with Peer Mental Health and the CEO of NewPath VR, now Newpath (Rizzo et al., 2021).

Virtual reality at USC: I've also been volunteering with the University of Southern California's Keck School of Medicine at the art gallery with Lyn Crandall, who the White House awarded for her outstanding volunteer work with the virtual reality gallery. Because the location at the Keck Medicine Campus gallery closed due to COVID, we developed a VR Gallery you can visit online and at Keck. (Please visit www. filmandvideoabsedtherapy.com to see a demonstration.)

Peer Mental Health is another project that I worked on while at a skilled nursing facility. I brought in one of the professors, Marlene Valter, who then worked with David Israelian to form a new psychological company. Dr. Valter, my assessments professor while I was getting my Ph.D. at Pacifica Graduate Institute, formed AnaVault as a separate company from Peer Mental Health due to some particularities in California law that didn't allow David Israelian to control the medical practice. I agree with that law, as getting a license is meant to protect the public. Peers should not influence it with mental health challenges or anyone not having the experience, education, and training. Later, the team at Peer Mental Health and AnaVault were discussed in my appearance on *Singularity Watch*. To see the broadcast, please visit https://filmandvideobasedtherapy.com. This podcast, *Virtual Reality (VR)*, was video recorded on an interview with Alt Space VR, where we had also done an in-person and virtual presentation back in 2020. It was presented before the COVID-19 pandemic as a collaborative effort between *VR* and a live audience at USC and later used different software in 2021 when the gallery opened again. To see both, please visit http://filmandvideobasedtherapy.com/.

In volume 2 of *Film/Video-Based Therapy*™ *and Trauma: Research and Practice*, we will discuss how filmmaking might utilize the gaming engine of the Unreal Engine to make films using Film/Video-Based Therapy™ and virtual reality.

Recently, Skip Rizzo interviewed film director and producer Brett Leonard, to explore these subjects (https://filmandvideobasedtherapy.com/; Cohen, 2022). With breakthrough technology from Lucasfilm and Disney for a TV show called *The Mandalorian* and a game developer in Egypt's Unreal Engine test, along with my introduction at NAB to the third-floor animation (also on the website https://filmandvideobasedtherapy.com/; Cohen, 2022), there are enough pieces to the puzzle to expand on in Volume 2 and still tell readers enough to understand the need for future research.

Also, there is a possibility of forming a collaboration with the military (https://filmandvideobasedtherapy.com/; Cohen, 2022) as both "I Was There" Films and the Institute of Creative Technologies worked with the Army and other servicemen and women on separate projects.

The previous book has a chapter written by Brian Austin (The animation Project) that outlines how to use art therapists in connection with animation. Peer Mental Health and CODIEPIE, David Israelian's other company, might play a role in future research. https:// filmandvideobasedtherapy.com/.

Conclusion

This work may involve technology and, in essence, the focus is still about highlighting psychological trauma and how one can cope with the over-whelming triggers in today's world. Therapy and Film/Video-Based Therapy™ should involve a licensed therapist, and, in the case of the work at Peer Mental Health and AnaVault, they have done that. The dif-ference is in separation of the clinical end. The people in the Czech Republic might see that keeping the therapist in the room might keep the clients safe; however, it restricts imagination and creativity in some cases. So doing assessments might help assist in fostering a therapeutic relation-ship, as Cathhy Malchiodi stated in her work (Cohen et al., 2015). In the future we will also focus, hopefully, on human potential and not the negative aspects of trauma but rather posttraumatic growth.

References

Anslow, J. A. (2012). Archetypes assemble: How superhero teams save the world from the apocalypse and lead the way to individuation—Marvel's *the Avengers*. *Spring Journal* 88: 233–246.

Cohen, J. L. (2019, 6). Call for abstracts – film/video-based therapy. Film/video-based therapy – from the book. *Video and Filmmaking as Psychotherapy: Research and Practice*. https://filmandvideobasedtherapy.com/2019/07/06/2019-7-5-call-for-abstracts/

Cohen, J. L. (2022, January 8). Film/Video-Based_Therapy_Website. www. filmandvideobasedtherapy.com

Cohen, J. L. (2021). *Home*. Film/video-based therapy. Retrieved September 11, 2022, from https://filmandvideobasedtherapy.com/2019/07/06/2019-7-5-call-for-abstracts/

Cohen, J. L., Johnson, J. L., & Orr, P. (2015). *Video and filmmaking as psycho-therapy: Research and practice*. Routledge.

Gartenberg, C. (2020, February 20). How the Mandalorian teamed up with Fortnite creator epic games to create its digital sets. *The Verge*. https://www.theverge.com/2020/2/20/21145671/mandalorian-sets-stagecraft-epic-games-ilm-fortnite-baby-yoda-digital

L.A. Castle Studios. (2020). L.A. Castle Studios. https://www.lacastlestudios.com/studio-updates/2020/2/20/the-mandalorian-shot-using-unreal-engine?gclid=CjwKCAjwieuGBhAsEiwA1Ly_nQIA6sJmAGq6YbyrFhMy6CG7UrVCsqi2AeVASDuBaRdXmNwVNXUHzhoCqUMQAvD_BwE

Levine, P. A. (1997). *Waking the tiger: Healing trauma: The innate capacity to transform overwhelming experiences*. North Atlantic Books.

Rizzo, A. (2022). Albert "Skip" Rizzo. Institute for Creative Technologies. https://ict.usc.edu/profile/albert-skip-rizzo/

Rizzo, A., Hartholt, A., & Mozgai, S. (2021). Establishment of clinical virtual reality methodologies from the front lines of Afghanistan to COVID-19. In: W. Greenleaf, L. Roberts, & R. Fine (Eds.), *Applied virtual reality in healthcare: Case studies and perspectives* (pp. 163–188). Cool Blue Media.

Rizzo, A. S. (2021, May 22). Podcast 02 Brett Leonard. *YouTube.* https://www. youtube.com/watch?v=vndMozRMOv8

Rogers, N. (2012). *The creative connection for groups.* Ohio University Center for International Studies.

Somatic Experiencing® International. (2021, November 9). About – Somatic Experiencing® International. https://traumahealing.org/about/

van der Kolk, B. A. (2015). *The body keeps the score: Brain, mind, and body in the healing of trauma.* Random House.

Wachowski, L. (2022). *The Matrix resurrections.* In theaters and on HBO Max December 22 | HBO Max. https://www.hbomax.com/the-matrix-resurrections-a?utm_id=sa%7c71700000086089950%7c58700007300197336%7cp6606 4587882&gclid=Cj0KCQiAieWOBhCYARIsANcOw0xbIudOa3jCEhvF025 QFsQI6mmMbU9T0krGaEaL05PfFr_UelCRYEQaAspnEALw_wcB& gclsrc=aw.ds

Part II

Trauma in the Home, City, State/Province

2 "No Longer under Water"

The Role of Metaphors in Trauma Re-Storying

Valentina Stoycheva

> I now believe that what therapists really do most of the time is (1) listen to people's stories, (2) help them to collaborate on a different narrative version that is more self-empowering, and (3) introduce stories in the form of metaphors, disclosures, modeling, and teaching tales.
>
> —Kottler (2017)

Traumatic events often bend the fabric of time and coherent narration, remaining etched in our memory in preverbal images and bodily sensations. How do we "unlock" them and put them into words to foster healing? Oftentimes, trauma therapists listen for what we call a "trauma narrative"— the story of a patient's experience of the traumatic event, its perceived causes, and its impact, which are frequently refracted through the lens of post-traumatic reexperiencing and cognitive alterations in the perception of self and the world. To take such a narrative and assist in recovery through the process of therapy, we must become familiar with the unconscious process of embodied cognition and how it relates to the formation of traumatic memories. "Re-storying" a traumatic event and its meaning for the survivor is a process that requires attunement to the ways in which the body responds to adverse events, knowledge of how thoughts are grounded in our physiology, and skill to translate physiological experiences back into words in a safe and holding environment. In this chapter, I review some of these processes and highlight the utility of metaphor-rich therapy in helping patients who contend with traumatic reactions feel seen and "gotten," and ultimately re-story their experiences in a way that facilitates meaning-making and integration into a more coherent narration of the self. Lastly, I also discuss how, through the use of metaphor, auxiliary therapies involving engagement of the sensory processing systems—e.g., visual and sensory-motor—could be valuable in transforming raw preverbal material into a narrative of healing.

Trauma is in the Body

In an unfortunate case of life imitates art, the scientific and psychological understanding of the profound impact of trauma arrived many centuries

DOI: 10.4324/9781315622507-4

after ancient scholars wrote about it in literary texts. Historical writings as old as 1,300BC–600BC (cf. Scurlock & Andersen, 2005) and better-known works by the Greek historian Herodotus and the poet Homer (*The Iliad* and *The Odyssey*) suggest that symptoms of what we today call post-traumatic stress disorder (PTSD) were known to humanity and recognizable to those who knew where to look millennia ago.

Post-traumatic stress disorder, however, did not appear as a diagnosis in the *Diagnostic and Statistical Manual of Mental Disorders* (DSM) until 1980 (*DSM-III*; American Psychiatric Association). After several decades of controversy and categorizing PTSD as an anxiety disorder, the *DSM* finally recognized traumatic responses as a discrete category of reactions—trauma- and stressor-related disorders—in its fifth incarnation (*DSM-5*; *American Psychiatric Association*, 2013). Our understanding of trauma and its sequelae has been evolving to include emotional regulation problems, hyperarousal and intrusive symptoms, and cognitive alterations. Only within the last decade have more popular works by Bessel van der Kolk (*The Body Keeps the Score*, 2014) and Peter Levine (*Healing Trauma*, 2008; *Trauma and Memory*, 2015) discussed the mechanisms through which trauma becomes "locked" in the body, perpetuating patterns of physiological activation and deactivation that impact virtually every aspect of our functioning, from physical illness to relationships with others, to proprioception. All the while, science is making headway in uncovering the potentially devastating impact of traumatic events on our physical health. Immunological responses related to PTSD in adults have been likened to the changes resulting from rheumatoid arthritis and multiple sclerosis, while sexual assault in adolescents has been found to cause dysregulations in the immune system functioning known to cause autoimmune diseases (Ayaydin et al., 2016).

Conversely, oxytocin (the connection hormone) has been found to lower the risk of developing PTSD after exposure to traumatic events (Frijling, 2017) and to show potential for augmenting trauma-focused psychotherapy (Flanagan et al., 2018; Koch et al., 2015). Not coincidentally, oxytocin has also been demonstrated to regulate immune function through performing an antibiotic-like function, promoting healing of wounds and tissue regeneration, and inhibiting inflammation and stress-related immune disorders (Li et al., 2017). The hormone largely produced when we feel connected appears to be quite literally physically healing us from within. It is no wonder, then, that researchers studying the effects of trauma have emphasized the effect of community and a sense of belonging as both a preventative factor and a factor facilitating the process of recovery (cf. Junger, 2016).

How the Body Reacts to Threat: Polyvagal Theory

Relatively recently, Dr. Steven Porges (1995, 2011) proposed what has become known as *the polyvagal theory*. Based on his studies of the connection between how our human nervous system evolved and the role of social engagement in emotional regulation, he was able to shed light on the links between physiological states and behavior. In particular, polyvagal theory explains what in the trauma literature is known as the fight-flight-freeze cycle of responses to traumatic events.

In studying the nervous system, Porges (2009, 2011) realized that the division of the nervous system into two branches—activating (sympathetic) and calming (parasympathetic)—is much more nuanced than previously thought. Specifically, there are separate neural mechanisms that govern social engagement, the fight-or-flight response, and the feign-death reaction (or what is today more commonly known as the freeze response). The three subsystems also originated at different times in our evolutionary development, with the freeze response being phylogenetically the oldest and the social-safety one being the newest.

According to polyvagal theory, when we are functioning optimally—i.e., when we are calm and connected—our parasympathetic nervous system is also appropriately regulating our engagement with the world, ensuring an ongoing sense of safety. We do not have to worry about our survival; therefore, we are free to fully focus on activities like goal-driven behavior and enjoyment. In a safe and social state, we are more in control of our reactions, we make thought-out choices, and feel overall comfortable and comforted in the presence of others even when stressors are present. However, when we experience significantly stressful and even life-threatening situations, we can quickly go down the ladder toward the two older mechanisms of coping: sympathetic activation (the fight/flight response) and parasympathetic lockdown (the freeze response). Biologically, this theory suggests, sympathetic activation comes first. In a dangerous situation, we are more likely to first try to escape or fight for survival. Only if those strategies prove unsuccessful do we experience a freeze response—overwhelming fatigue or fainting, immobility, or psychological dissociation.

As psychologists, we often witness patients working through trauma in our office experience fight, flight, or freeze reactions. Even the memory of a traumatic event can be a powerful trigger for sympathetic activation or parasympathetic lock to occur. It is not uncommon for a patient to become very emotionally activated or dissociated in session, due to reexperiencing or flashbacks of the trauma that brought them to therapy in the first place. Importantly, once fight, flight, or freeze have been established as well-rehearsed responses to any type of danger—real or perceived, physical or emotional—a person is likely to automatically use them, whether or not the environment is in fact safe. For a survivor of violence in childhood, for example, an angry facial expression may be sufficient to cause a freeze response (emotional shutdown, dissociation). This is particularly relevant to treatment, which can often be experienced as emotionally threatening even by the most motivated patient due to, by its nature, forcing the individual to work through very painful experiences, memories, and emotions. It behooves us as therapists to learn how to create the safe environment that our patients need to help them process painful experiences in a way that allows them to exit fight/flight/freeze responses and restore functioning in the safe and social position, which, in turn, ensures flexibility in their utilization of coping and regulatory strategies. Metaphors can provide one such avenue of expediting a feeling of connectedness but to understand how they can assist us in this endeavor, we must first learn about embodied cognition. As we shall see, it is not only emotional responses that are grounded in our bodies; it is also thoughts and, by extension, communication and narration.

Embodied Cognition

The theoretical proposition that our thoughts are grounded in our physiology is relatively new. It can be somewhat dated back to William James's (1890) discussion of emotions, in which he proposed that the realization of experiencing emotions comes after the bodily reaction they engender (e.g., we are afraid because we run, not the other way around), but it was not until the last few decades that the phenomenon of embodied cognition has garnered significant empirical support. The essence of embodied cognition is deceptively simple—cognitive states are embedded in the body (embodied). Every thought, opinion, and judgment we form, conscious or unconscious, is in some way grounded in the physiology of our body. In turn, our experience of and within our bodies impacts our thoughts and perceptions of ourselves and the world. This has important implications for understanding how our minds use metaphors (grasping one concept through the use of another) for understanding our reality.

A growing body of research has unequivocally demonstrated that embodied cognition holds true: the mind is grounded in our body's physical interactions with the world. Our cognitive states are often, if not always, rooted in our orientation in time and space, as well as in sensory experiences. Several lines of inquiry in the sensory domains of temperature, taste, time, and space have demonstrated this. In a series of experiments, Williams and Bargh (2008) demonstrated that when an experimenter handed study participants a cup of warm liquid, the participants rated the experimenter as "warmer" (personality trait) than participants who had been handed a cold beverage. Similarly, in a second experiment, participants who held a warm therapeutic pad, as opposed to the control group who held a cold one, engaged in pro-social behavior significantly more frequently. Sensory perception of warmth, then, is related to social judgments and behaviors. Further, in another study (Zhong & Leonardelli, 2008), researchers found that individuals who are prompted to remember a social inclusion situation rated the room temperature as significantly higher than individuals who recalled instances of feeling excluded. Quite literally, feeling connected makes us feel "warm and fuzzy," while loneliness feels cold.

Another dimension of human experience, taste, is also powerfully implicated in how cognitions are formed. If you have ever wondered why some people are judged as "sweet" and others as "bitter," when in fact we do not actually taste them, this is why. Perception of taste is a marker through which we orient ourselves in the world; similarly, this sensory experience is used to navigate our social worlds. And this transposition is also based on physiology. Meier et al. (2012) demonstrated that study participants who savored a candy or a piece of chocolate not only rated themselves as more agreeable but also spontaneously engaged in more uncompensated helpful behaviors when compared to a control group who did not taste a sweet treat. They tasted something sweet and then *acted* sweetly! Conversely, bitterness has been associated with hostility. Sagioglu and Greitemeyer (2014) demonstrated that participants who were asked to consume a bitter beverage subsequently showed an increase in self-reported hostility, aggressive affect, and angry behavior.

Growing evidence suggests that even our perceptions of time and space are embodied, with time as a more abstract concept being highly dependent on our orientation in space as a proxy. In a rather clever experiment, Boroditsky and Ramscar (2002) demonstrated that manipulating an object to move either forward or backward primed participants with these concepts, resulting in changing their perception of time. After viewing the object move, the participants read the sentence "Next Wednesday's meeting has been moved forward two days" (p. 186). The group who saw an object move backward guessed that the new day for the meeting would be Monday, while the group who witnessed an object being moved forward guessed that the new meeting day would be Friday. In a second experiment, the researchers demonstrated that the results held true if people themselves were asked to move forward or backward in a line.

These, and many other studies, demonstrate that to grasp complex concepts (like time), our minds defer to concepts that we can physically relate to (like space). We do this automatically and unconsciously, without awareness. Moreover, Gilead et al. (2015) confirmed that the embodiment of cognition is a normative process that takes place across cultures. It is not surprising, then, that if so much of our typical day-to-day functioning is embedded in our bodies, extraordinary experiences that shake up our world, and us within it, will also have significant physiological correlates. Embodiment also provides a level of understanding of how our physiological reactions to trauma (fight/flight/freeze) may become narratives, impacting heavily how we tell our story of the experience and ourselves in it, as well as subsequent ways of viewing ourselves and the world. Metaphors, on the other hand, seem like an effective translator, a Babel fish if you like, of our innermost hard-to-verbalize experiences into language.

The Role of Metaphors

There is a saying, attributed to the Asaro tribe of Papua New Guinea, which states, "Knowledge is only a rumor until it lives in the muscle" (as cited in Brown, 2015, p. 7). A number of years ago, one of my patients created her own version of this saying. In re-narrating her childhood trauma from a story of self-blame and shame to one of resilience, she stated, "I have this new insight now, but I still need to make it part of my cells."

Making new knowledge part of our cells is exactly where, I believe, embodiment, polyvagal theory, and metaphors converge in trauma therapy. Paying attention to metaphors in psychotherapy dates back to psychoanalysis and Freud (1900), but only recently have we become better equipped to understand their utility more fully and through relying on more empirically supported lines of inquiry such as embodied cognition. Martin et al. (1992) demonstrated that patients remember therapist-introduced metaphors at a rate higher than chance (two-thirds of the time) and that the sessions in which those metaphors were used were perceived by patients as significantly more helpful than sessions in which patients did not recall metaphors. More importantly, when asked why they perceived metaphors as helpful, the patients reported that metaphors not only increased their emotional insight and clarified their goals but also enhanced their connection with the therapist.

Metaphors as a tool in therapy have the capacity to resolve paradox and foster new learning which would have been impossible by merely describing experience. They evoke feelings, images, and concepts—as well as relationships between the three—which may have previously been hidden from awareness and thus inaccessible to verbalization. Even more importantly, I believe, they provide a means of connecting and sharing one's innermost experience in a way that allows another human being to enter into our very idiosyncratic universe. In therapy, it is only through entering this very private narration of the trauma memory that therapists are able to help their patients shift and re-story their experience.

From an embodied cognition framework, there are two possible explanations about why metaphors have such an impact (cf. Weinberger & Stoycheva, 2019). The first one relies on environmental pairing of concepts. Take the metaphor of affection as warmth, for example. We learn to equate warmth with affection at infancy, when we are comforted by a hopefully patient and loving caregiver. Hugs are physically warm and emotionally comforting; therefore, warmth becomes a proxy for comfort. The second-proposed mechanism of embodiment is evolutionary in nature. It is an implication of the process of exaptation—the utilization of an older bodily or brain structure for an evolutionarily new purpose. According to this theory, which has significant empirical support (Anderson, 2010, 2014; Dehaene, 2005; Gallese, 2007; Gallese & Lakoff,

2005), brain neurons which originally evolved for motor and sensory activity later became co-opted for cognitive and emotional-regulatory functions. Therefore, the brain regions that are activated when we think of physical comfort are the same regions tasked with warmth perception. Similarly, it is possible that brain regions responsible for space perception have been exapted to help us understand the much more complex concept of time.

Clinical support for these proposed mechanisms of work of metaphors comes from studying how patients discuss traumatic events. Tay and Jordan (2015), for example, interviewed survivors of the 2010–2012 earthquakes in New Zealand and found that the most common language that the interviewees used to describe their experience was metaphorical. Both physical/concrete loss and a feeling of loss of control were frequently expressed through abstract language, using metaphors like "sitting at the back of a jumbo jet…not being able to get a hold" of loved ones. Loss of interpersonal contact was quickly replaced by a feeling of loss of anchors. Another participant used the expression "the whole ground had shifted" (Tay & Jordan, 2015, p. 562) to convey an overwhelming sense of uncertainty about the future, and still another described the aftermath of an earthquake in terms of its long-lasting psychological impact stating, "the ground was still moving" and "we were in the dark" (Tay & Jordan, 2015, p. 563).

These metaphors of powerful seismic shifts in people's perception of themselves, and the world around them reflect trauma survivors' experience in a very powerful way. They are similar to my own experience as a trauma therapist and my own patients' attempts at making sense of their experience. One patient described herself as a "rescue truck"—always on standby, unable to ever relax, putting out the fires (also a metaphor) in her loved ones' lives. Another spoke of horrific childhood abuse by naming her family situation "The Texas Chainsaw Massacre." Yet another childhood sexual assault survivor described her daily experiences as being "under water"—muted, dulled, and blurry—much like her memories of the original trauma. For this patient, the subjective perception of being under water reflected a sense of disconnect from the world, an experience of dissociation and fear of being fully present. It further signified the fractured, unreal quality of her memories, which had initially led to doubting them in the first place—to doubting her own narrative of the trauma. Through sharing this metaphor, she allowed me to enter this underwater world with her. In doing so, she was no longer alone in it, and, as a result, her parasympathetic nervous system did not automatically enter into a lockdown (dissociative state). This way, I was able to assist her in gaining more clarity, processing the importance of acknowledging the realness of the memories, and eventually experiencing the world and herself in it as real again. "No longer under water," she was able to own her story and even expressed a wish to write it as the next step of her post-traumatic growth.

These findings, empirical and anecdotal, are particularly notable in our understanding of how metaphors in therapy are healing—they may be the vehicle through which we embody new knowledge in a safe and social physiological state. It is possible that in-session metaphors, through helping the patient feel "seen" and "gotten," reinstate a sense of safety, deactivate the fight-flight and death-feigning responses, and assist individuals in processing their traumatic memories without the powerful and overwhelming reexperiencing reactions that take place when trauma memories are elicited in an uncontained environment. Metaphorical language invites the therapist into the patient's world in a way that ordinary description cannot, thus allowing the patient to feel less alone in the terrifying and lonely place of trauma. Thus, metaphors not only "shake up" our old narratives and help create new, more adaptive, ones, but also facilitate doing so while in a state of connectedness with a warm and supportive other who is capable of soothing our hyperactivated nervous system through making us feel seen at our core.

Art Imitating Life for Healing

Metaphors, in connecting bodily experiences with language to foster healing, may also hold the key to why a growing number of studies are finding that technology-assisted auxiliary treatments may be helpful in trauma recovery (cf. Cohen & Orr, 2015). While this field is still in its infancy, a 2018 qualitative study by Tuval-Mashiach et al. (2018) found that when veterans created short artistic films that reflected on their military experience, they reported subjective positive impact on regaining a sense of agency and affiliation, as well as on reworking their trauma narratives. Video-based interventions, the authors argue, may be able to tap into the physicality of traumatic memories through accessing sensory, not-yet-verbalized, information. Through the use of metaphors, the films are then able to translate this information into a new narrative of the traumatic experiences.

Also, in addressing combat PTSD in the past decade or so, traveling Theatre of War productions have brought many a veteran and civilian to tears with their dramatic readings of ancient Greek plays. In a 2016 *New Yorker* profile, the founder and director of the productions, Bryan Doerries, admits that it took numerous performances before he realized that people want to discuss the shadowy side of humanity, later reflecting on the connective function that performances of tragedy have on the audience (Wright, 2016). Through art and metaphor, we are able to dress in words that which has, up to that point, been unspeakable—locked and frozen in the body—and metabolize it in safety. As discussed earlier, polyvagal theory explains how shared experience (in this case, for the audience) provides the safety in which traumatic material may be brought up and reprocessed while the individual experiences themselves in a safe and social state, rather than a fight/flight/freeze state.

In working with a veteran from the early Iraq invasions several years ago, I distinctly remember the physiological activation and hypervigilance notable in the room at first. Based on his report, they were mirrored by significant agitation during driving. Overseas, he said, he had not been allowed to stop or slow down even in populated areas because of the risk of an ambush—a way of driving completely unsuitable for functioning in a suburban landscape full of stop signs and school buses. In addition, he had a difficult time driving under overpasses or passing garbage pails, which triggered intense bouts of panic related to the fear of explosions, which had been common in theater. Through finally being able to talk about his trauma and re-story his experiences overseas into a more coherent narrative, this veteran became gradually able to separate past from present and become better able to modulate his emotional responses to perceived triggers. Many metaphors were used throughout his treatment, but perhaps the most poignant one was of him describing how, though reworking and integrating the trauma in the safety of the therapeutic office (and relationship), he had been able to "switch to neutral gear." Finally, he shared at the end of treatment, he was able to relax and establish a sense of safety—in driving and in living in general.

In Conclusion

Traumatic events can oftentimes leave a person without words to describe what has happened to them or their experiences resulting from the trauma. This is not uncommon, due to the significant somatic and physiological reactions that trauma induces in our bodies—reactions for which we often do not have the necessary language. Trauma becomes embedded in the body, causing significant disruptions to our emotional, cognitive, and relational worlds. Metaphors, as a vehicle for accessing unverbalized experiences and giving them shape, can be particularly useful in healing from trauma. They allow the person not only to narrate their experience in a way which may not have otherwise been possible but also to feel seen and understood through the shared knowledge of the metaphor's meaning. This mutual process of sharing and receiving sensitive information can foster a sense of safety, in which the individual can reprocess and re-narrate their experiences. It behooves us as psychologists, counselors, and social workers to better understand the role and use of metaphors, as well as the forms of art which use them—such as film, video, narrative storytelling—and explore ways of incorporating them in our work.

References

American Psychiatric Association. (1980). *Diagnostic and statistical manual of mental disorders* (3rd ed.). Author.

American Psychiatric Association. (2013). *Diagnostic and statistical manual of mental disorders* (5th ed.). Author. doi: 10.1176/appi.books.9780890425596

Anderson, M. L. (2010). Neural reuse: A fundamental organisational principle of the brain. *Behavioural and Brain Sciences, 33*(4), 245–266. doi: 10.1017/S0140525X10000853

Anderson, M. L. (2014). *After phrenology: Neural reuse and the interactive brain.* MIT Press.

Ayaydin, H., Abali, O., Akdeniz, N. O., Kok, B. E., Gunes, A., Yildirim, A., & Deniz, G. (2016). Immune system changes after sexual abuse in adolescents. *Pediatrics International, 58*(2), 105–112. doi: 10.1111/ped.12767. PMID: 26224367.

Boroditsky, L., & Ramscar, M. (2002). The roles of body and mind in abstract thought. *Psychological Science, 13*(2), 185–189. doi: 10.1111/1467-9280.00434

Brown, B. (2015). *Daring greatly: How the courage to be vulnerable transforms the way we live, love, parent, and lead.* Avery.

Cohen, J. L., & Orr, P. P. (2015). Film/video-based therapy and editing as process from a depth psychological perspective. In J. L. Cohen, J. L. Johnson, & P. P. Orr. (Eds.), *Video and filmmaking as psychotherapy: Research and practice* (pp. 29–42). Routledge.

Dehaene, S. (2005). Evolution of human cortical circuits for reading and arithmetic: The "neuronal recycling" hypothesis. In S. Dehaene, J. R. Duhamen, M. D. Hauser, & G. Rizolatti (Eds.), *From monkey brain to human brain* (pp. 133–157). MIT Press.

Flanagan, J. C., Sippel, L. M., Wahlquist, A., Moran-Santa Maria, M. M., & Back, S. E. (2018). Augmenting prolonged exposure therapy for PTSD with intranasal oxytocin: A randomized, placebo-controlled pilot trial. *Journal of Psychiatric Research, 98*, 64–69. doi: 10.1016/j.jpsychires.2017.12.014

Freud, S. (1900). *The interpretation of dreams.* Franz Deuticke.

Frijling, J. L. (2017). Preventing PTSD with oxytocin: Effects of oxytocin administration on fear neurocircuitry and PTSD symptom development in recently trauma-exposed individuals. *European Journal of Psychotraumatology, 8*(1), Article 1302652. doi: 10.1080/20008198.2017.1302652

Gallese, V. (2007). Before and below 'theory of mind': Embodied simulation and the neural correlates of social cognition. *Philosophical Transactions of the Royal Society B: Biological Sciences, 362*(1480), 659–669. doi: 10.1098/rstb.2006.2002

Gallese, V., & Lakoff, G. (2005). The brain's concepts: The role of the sensory-motor system in conceptual knowledge. *Cognitive Neuropsychology, 22*(3–4), 455–479. doi: 10.1080/02643290442000310

Gilead, M., Gal, O., Polak, M., & Cholow, Y. (2015). The role of nature and nurture in conceptual metaphors: The case of gustatory priming. *Social Psychology, 46*, 167–173. doi: 10.1027/1864-9335/a000238

James, W. (1890). *The principles of psychology* (Vols 1 & 2). Holt.

Junger, S. (2016). *Tribe: On homecoming and belonging.* Hachette.

Koch, S. B. J., van Zuiden, M., Nawijn, L., Frijling, J. L., Veltman, D. J., & Olff, M. (2015). Intranasal oxytocin administration dampens amygdala reactivity towards emotional faces in male and female PTSD patients. *Neuropsychopharmacology, 41*(6), 1495–1504. doi: 10.1038/npp.2015.299

Kottler, J. (2017). *On being a therapist* (5th ed.). Oxford University Press.

Levine, P. A. (2008). *Healing trauma: A pioneering program for restoring the wisdom of your body.* Sounds True.

Levine, P. A. (2015). *Trauma and memory: Brain and body in a search for the living past: A practical guide for understanding and working with traumatic memory*. North Atlantic Books.

Li, T., Wang, P., Wang, S., & Wang. Y. (2017). Approaches mediating oxytocin regulation of the immune system. *Frontiers in Immunology, 7*, 693. doi: 10.3389/fimmu.2016.00693

Martin, J., Cummings, A. L., & Hallberg, E. T. (1992). Therapists' intentional use of metaphor: Memorability, clinical impact, and possible epistemic/motivational functions. *Journal of Consulting and Clinical Psychology, 60*(1), 143–145. doi: 10.1037/0022-006X.60.1.143

Meier, B. P., Moeller, S. K., Riemer-Peltz, M., & Robinson, M. D. (2012). Sweet taste preferences and experiences predict prosocial inferences, personalities, and behaviors. *Journal of Personality and Social Psychology, 102*(1), 163–174. doi: 10.1037/a0025253

Porges, S. (1995). Orienting in a defensive world: Mammalian modifications of our evolutionary heritage: A polyvagal theory. *Psychophysiology, 32*, 301–318.

Porges, S. (2009). The polyvagal theory: New insights into adaptive reactions of the autonomic nervous system. *Cleveland Clinic Journal of Medicine, 76*(Suppl 2), S86–S90.

Porges, S. (2011). *Polyvagal theory: Neurophysiological foundations of emotions, attachment, communication, and self-regulation*. W. W. Norton.

Sagioglu, C., & Greitemeyer, T. (2014). Facebook's emotional consequences: Why Facebook causes a decrease in mood and why people still use it. *Computers in Human Behavior, 35*, 359–363. doi: 10.1016/j.chb.2014.03.003

Scurlock, J. A., & Andersen, B. R. (2005). *Diagnoses in Assyrian and Babylonian medicine: Ancient sources, translations, and modern medical analyses*. University of Illinois Press.

Tay, D., & Jordan, J. (2015). Metaphor and the notion of control in trauma talk. *Text & Talk, 35*(4), 553–573. doi: 10.1515/text-2015-0009

Tuval-Mashiach, R., Patton, B. W., & Drebing, C. (2018). "When you make a movie, and you see your story there, you can hold it": Qualitative exploration of collaborative filmmaking as a therapeutic tool for veterans. *Frontiers in Psychology, 9*. doi: 10.3389/fpsyg.2018.01954

van der Kolk, B. (2014). *The body keeps the score: Brain, mind, and body in the healing of trauma*. Viking.

Weinberger, J., & Stoycheva, V. (2019). *The unconscious: Theory, research, and clinical implications*. Guilford.

Williams, L. E., & Bargh, J. A. (2008). Experiencing physical warmth promotes interpersonal warmth. *Science, 322*(5901), 606–607. doi: 10.1126/science.1162548

Wright, R. (2016, September 12). Theatre of war: Sophocles' message for American veterans. *The New Yorker*. https://www.newyorker.com/culture/culture-desk/theatre-of-war-sophocles-message-for-american-veterans

Zhong, C.-B., & Leonardelli, G. J. (2008). Cold and lonely: Does social exclusion literally feel cold? *Psychological Science, 19*(9), 838–842. doi: 10.1111/j.1467-9280.2008.02165.x

3 The Application of Neurocinematics within Trauma Therapies and Integrative Practices

Bronwyn Robertson

Introduction

The application of neuroscience within psychotherapy has become a mainstay of effective trauma therapies and evidence-based practices (Cozolino, 2010; Siegel, 2010; van der Kolk, 2004). This chapter explores how a specific branch of neuroscience, neurocinematics, can be effectively and ethically applied within trauma therapy. Neurocinematics, the neuroscientific study of film and cinema, has been widely used by filmmakers and consumer scientists (Hasson et al., 2008). When ethically applied within psychotherapy, neurocinematic research and techniques can enhance trauma treatment. This author will highlight case studies utilizing neurocinematics in Trauma-Focused Cognitive-Behavior Therapy (TF-CBT) and mindfulness-based, expressive and Somatic Experiencing (SE) practices and protocols for acute and complex post-traumatic stress, secondary trauma, and traumatic grief.

The utilization of neuroscientific research within psychotherapy has led to the development of some of the most effective trauma therapies and integrative practices (Cozolino, 2010, 2017; Siegel, 2009, 2010; Van der Kolk, 2000; Welton & Kay, 2015). For more than a quarter century, research from the affective and cognitive neurosciences has been instrumental in advancing our understanding of what is effective in the psychotherapeutic treatment of trauma. Most recently, the information and techniques gleaned from the neuroscientific study of cinema, or neurocinematics, are showing promise when directly applied within the therapeutic treatment of trauma via cinematherapy (Robertson, 2016).

According to Welton and Kay (2015), advancements in neuroscience, specifically in neuroimaging techniques, led to the neurobiological understanding of "what happens in the brain when the mind is engaged in psychotherapy" (Welton and Kay, 2015, section 1). Van der Kolk (2000) similarly credits the role of neuroimaging studies in enhancing the neurobiological understanding of trauma and the development of new, integrative trauma therapies:

DOI: 10.4324/9781315622507-5

Developments in the neurosciences have started to make significant contributions to our understanding of how the brain is shaped by experience....The study of trauma has probably been the single most fertile area within the disciplines of psychiatry and psychology in helping to develop a deeper understanding of the interrelationships between emotional, cognitive, social, and biological forces that shape human development. Research in these areas has opened up entirely new insights in how extreme experiences throughout the life cycle can have profound effects on memory, affect regulation, biological stress modulation, and interpersonal relatedness. These findings, in the context of the development of a range of new therapy approaches, are beginning to open up entirely new perspectives on how traumatized individuals can be helped to overcome their past.

(p. 19)

Integrative Approaches to Trauma Therapy

Recognized leaders in the research and treatment of trauma—Peter Levine, Dan Siegel, and Bessel van der Kolk—have all pioneered integrative approaches to trauma treatment based on neuroscience. Their work supports the premise that integrative psychotherapy promotes neurobiological integration which is essential for effective trauma treatment.

Levine began developing the Somatic Experiencing (SE) approach to trauma treatment more than 45 years ago. This approach views trauma as long-term dysregulation in the body, brain, and nervous system. Somatic Experiencing focuses on bringing body, or somatic, awareness into the psychotherapeutic process by primarily focusing on clients' physiological sensations rather than just their cognitive or emotional experiences. As noted by Payne et al. (2015), "unlike conventional psychotherapy which focuses largely on verbal cognitive processes, the focus of SE is on the functioning of the deeper, regulatory, levels of the nervous system, in particular the autonomic nervous system (ANS) ... and the limbic system" (p. 2).

Siegel, recognized for his work in interpersonal neurobiology and creator of the Mindsight approach to psychotherapy, sees the therapist's role as helping clients integrate their body, brain, and mind. Siegel's Mindsight (2009) uses mindfulness practices and techniques to enhance "internal attunement" and integration. To Siegel, mental health is based on integration, which "leads to flexible, adaptive, and coherent flow of energy and information in the brain, the mind, and relationships" (p. 137).

Van der Kolk began his award-winning neuroscientific research of traumatic stress in the 1970s and has published extensively on the subject ever since. His research has shown that "the brain's natural ability to integrate experience breaks down" in individuals who have posttraumatic stress disorder (van der Kolk, 2006, p. 12). According to van der

Kolk (2006), interoceptive, body-oriented therapies can, among other things, directly address a core clinical issue in trauma-related disorders: "Traumatized individuals are prone to experience the present with physical sensations and emotions from the past" (p. 13). He has also noted that it is more useful for therapists "to focus on the patient's physical self-experience and increase their self-awareness, rather than focusing exclusively on the meaning that people make of their experience—their narrative of the past" (p. 13). For van der Kolk (2005), the treatment of trauma, especially complex or developmental trauma, needs to focus on the integration of the body and brain to be effective.

The experience of trauma at any time during one's lifespan can disrupt integration among neural networks in the brain, according to Cozolino (2010). Early childhood or complex trauma is particularly damaging, however, and "can cause ongoing information processing deficits that disrupt integrated neural processing" throughout the lifespan (p. 24).

Brain imaging and electroencephalography (EEG) studies show that normal brain functioning requires the integration and synchronization of specific neural networks within the brain (Uhlhaas & Singer, 2006). In "The Neuroscience of Psychotherapy," Cozolino (2010) defines psychotherapy as a means of enhancing or restoring the functioning and integration of neural networks. Successful psychotherapy, according to Cozolino, actually activates areas of the brain associated with symptoms of mental health disorders and promotes "repeated simultaneous activation of networks requiring integration with one another" (p. 25).

As Siegel (2009) noted, the brain's medial prefrontal cortex (mPFC) is the center of integration within the brain and body and "connects everything together" (p. 143). Neuroimaging studies show that the mPFC is among the main areas in the brain directly affected by traumatic stress (van der Kolk, 2000). According to van der Kolk (2006), psychotherapy must activate the same areas of the brain which are impacted by traumatic stress to effectively treat trauma:

> Neurobiologically speaking, they [clients] need to activate their mPFC (medial prefrontal cortex), insula, and anterior cingulate by learning to tolerate orienting and focusing their attention on their internal experience, while interweaving and conjoining cognitive, emotional, and sensorimotor elements of their traumatic experience.
> (p. 12)

The Neuroscience of Trauma

Neuroimaging studies have shown that traumatic stress can alter functioning in specific areas of the brain, disrupt activation of neural circuits, and reduce integration, connectivity and synchrony in neural networks which mediate the stress response and fear conditioning responses

(Blechert et al., 2007; Simon & Engström, 2015; van der Kolk, 2004, 2006). Research has also established that these brain changes are associated with specific symptoms of posttraumatic stress disorder (PTSD) (Sherin & Nemeroff, 2011; van der Kolk, 2006). Welton and Kay (2015) noted that "learning to be afraid," or fear conditioning, is a process which involves interactions in the mPFC, amygdala, insula, and the anterior cingulate cortex (ACC). Fear extinction, or the process of unlearning fear, is central to many trauma therapies and requires normal, unaltered functioning in the mPFC, ACC, and hippocampus.

Brain imaging studies of individuals with PTSD show altered functioning in the mPFC, prefrontal cortex (PFC), ACC, insula, and main structures in the limbic system including the hippocampus and amygdala (Sherin & Nemeroff, 2011). For example, heightened activation of structures within the mPFC and the limbic system is associated with intrusive symptoms such as flashbacks (Cozolino, 2010). Severity of PTSD symptoms is linked to increased activation in the ACC, whereas decreased activation of the ACC is associated with the extinction of conditioned fear responses (Sherin & Nemeroff, 2011; Uhlhaas & Singer, 2006).

Neuroimaging research also links core PTSD symptoms such as intrusions, reexperiencing, avoidance, and hyperarousal to dysfunction within the brain's default mode network (DMN) (Sherin & Nemeroff, 2011; Simon & Engström, 2015). The main structures involved in the DMN include the PFC, mPFC, ACC, and amygdala. DMN activation is associated with a resting brain state and includes autobiographical memory, self-related processing, mind wandering, envisioning future events, empathy, and social processing (Parker & Razlighi, 2019; Simon & Engström, 2015). Neuroscience research shows that mindfulness practices have a positive effect on the functioning of the DMN and are associated with a resting brain state (Simon & Engström, 2015), whereas the impact of traumatic stress impairs its functioning and is associated with PTSD symptom severity (Akiki et al., 2018; Viard et al., 2019).

One of the first neuroimaging studies of individuals with PTSD was conducted by van der Kolk and associates in 1996 (Rauch et al., 1996). In this study, individuals were exposed to vivid and detailed accounts of their own traumatic experiences via a script which they read while undergoing a positron emission tomography (PET) brain scan (van der Kolk, 2000). The purpose of this study was to explore the neuroanatomy of PTSD symptoms by measuring brain changes in individuals with PTSD while they were in a symptomatic state. The study involved both triggering and measuring PTSD symptoms. Van der Kolk (2000) has noted that the results showed decreased activation in the left inferior frontal area of the brain while individuals were reading their trauma scripts. This area is associated with the ability to translate and communicate personal experiences via language.

Many cognitive and affective neuroimaging studies involve the use of scripts, movies, videos, and animation in the study of trauma. Nixon et al. (2007), for example, measured intrusive memories in individuals diagnosed with PTSD by showing them films of traumatic content during neuroimaging studies. Similarly, Rombold-Bruehl et al. (2018) used films depicting severe physical and sexual violence to measure memory impairment via neuroimaging studies in individuals who had experienced traumatic events.

Cinema is a powerful medium and is a "useful tool to study human affective neuroscience" (Cha et al., 2015, p. 186). As noted by Campbell et al. (2015), movies, videos, and animation "have the power to transport your mind from the narrow, impersonal bore of [a] magnetic resonance imaging (MRI) magnet to a world more synonymous with everyday life, replete with sights, sounds and language" (p. 3045). While cinema has proven useful in the study and assessment of trauma-related disorders, it also has the potential to enhance trauma therapy.

Neurocinematics

More than four decades of research have shown that cinematherapy, the therapeutic use of films, TV shows, videos, and animation, is effective in the treatment of a wide range of mental health challenges and disorders (Cohen et al., 2015). International studies have shown that cinematherapy can be effectively integrated into the psychotherapeutic treatment of anxiety and trauma-related disorders in varying age groups in multiple settings (Lorusso & Venturini, 2020; Robertson, 2016).

The neuroscientific study of cinema, or neurocinematics, uses neuroimaging techniques such as functional magnetic resonance imaging (fMRI), magnetoencephalography (MEG), and positron emission tomography, along with electroencephalography (EEG) and neurophysiological measures such as galvanic skin response and eye tracking, to monitor viewers' responses to specific selections of cinema, video, and animation. Neurocinematic studies can record moment-by-moment changes in viewers' brain functioning and neurophysiology while they are watching selected segments of cinema and establish which areas of the brain and nervous system are being activated or deactivated (Kaltwasser et al., 2019). Neurocinematic research also shows that specific cinematic techniques can direct and maintain viewers' attention, enhance neural synchrony and integration, evoke cognitive, emotional, and physiological responses, and even activate the same areas of the brain impacted by traumatic stress (Cha et al., 2015; Hasson et al., 2008; van der Kolk, 2006).

The neurocinematic branch of neuroscience was pioneered by Princeton University neuroscientist Uri Hasson in the early 2000s (Hasson et al., 2004, 2008). Hasson's studies established that cinema provides viewers with multisensory experiences measurable via neurocinematic imaging techniques (Hasson et al., 2008). Raz and Hendler (2014) have also noted the ability of movies to "hijack" the viewer's physiological systems and generate "powerful engagement with fictional characters" (p. 89). Similarly, Kaltwasser et al. (2019) have explained how the cinema connects with viewers on an embodied level when they identify "with onscreen characters." It can induce a range of physiological and neurophysiological responses including alterations in physiological processes associated with emotional arousal such as galvanic skin response (GSR), respiratory sinus arrhythmia (RSA), vagal activity, and the autonomic nervous system:

> As the multisensory experience of film can induce a wide range of affective responses, several studies have used film clips, especially those with an intense emotional content, to investigate the physiological reactions of the Autonomic Nervous System (ANS) to emotions. This greater capability in inducing physiological reactions is related to several advantages that movies have in comparison to other emotion-inducing methods.
>
> (p. 2)

Applying Neurocinematics to Psychotherapy

While much research has been done on the utilization of neuroscience and the integration of cinematherapy within psychotherapy, very little has been published which connects the two via neurocinematics. Only a handful of publications have explored specific applications of neurocinematic research and techniques in the field of psychotherapy (Lorusso & Venturini, 2020). What has been published suggests that the use of neurocinematics can augment diagnosis and assessment and enhance psychotherapy (Robertson, 2016; Schultebraucks et al., 2019; Sonkusare et al., 2019).

"All things connect: The Integration of Mindfulness, Cinema and Psychotherapy" is the first known publication by a psychotherapist which references the therapeutic application of neurocinematics within psychotherapy (Robertson, 2016). The article explores this author's application of mindfulness-oriented cinematherapy and neurocinematics in group therapy with more than 1,000 adults diagnosed with varying mental health disorders. As noted in the article, clients were better able to learn and practice mindfulness-based relaxation and self-regulation skills after viewing specific cinematic selections in group sessions.

In the article, the use of a specific television episode—"all things" from *The X-files* series (Anderson, 2000)—was highlighted and reported as having "remarkable results" in group therapy sessions. The 45-minute episode explores themes such as personal transformation, synchronicity, and concepts of mindfulness and mind-body connection. This author found it very useful in introducing concepts and practices of mindfulness to individuals who had little or no prior exposure, and who were in need of basic mindfulness skills to manage anxiety, mood, and trauma-related symptoms. Mindfulness practices have been found effective in decreasing trauma-related symptoms such as dissociation, dysregulation, and avoidance (Baer et al., 2006). Studies have also shown that mindfulness practices enhance empathy (Dekeyser et al., 2008), positive affect, optimism, and life satisfaction (Brown & Ryan, 2003).

In 90-minute to 2-hour group sessions, clients were guided through mindfulness practices before and/or after watching the episode and given time to share and process their experiences. As measured via client self-report, various assessments, and clinical observation, clients were noted as becoming much calmer, less reactive, and/or more reflective immediately after viewing the episode. For example, more than 100 clients reported being able to shift out of highly anxious or agitated states into calmer, more reflective states while viewing the episode. Most clients readily engaged while watching the episode, were able to process their experiences of the episode immediately after watching it and complete more in-depth exploration via homework assignments such as mindfulness exercises, journaling, poetry, writing life scripts, making artwork, and composing music. Only a handful of more than 1,000 clients did not complete their homework.

The episode was regularly used in group therapy for trauma survivors, with positive results. Clients reported that watching the episode in a group session and completing their homework assignments helped them safely identify and begin processing traumatic experiences. At least ten clients contacted this author two or more years after they completed group therapy to report continued progress in managing trauma-related symptoms via the mindfulness concepts and skills learned in the group sessions.

Neurocinematics, Trauma Therapy, and Integrative Practices

This author has suggested that the way the "all things" episode was directed and filmed produced a calming, mindfulness-inducing effect on clients, and may have even stimulated neural synchrony and bilateral stimulation. The evidenced-based trauma treatment eye movement desensitization and reprocessing (EMDR) is known to produce bilateral stimulation, for example. As described in "The Neurobiology of Eye Movement Desensitization and Reprocessing" by Vojtová and Hašto (2009), EMDR produces bilateral stimulation via sensory stimuli which "alternately elicit left and right hemispheric activity through visual, tactile or auditory modalities" (p. 98). Research suggests that bilateral stimulation, along with procedural elements such as "mindfulness-like attitude" and somatic awareness, enhances the therapeutic effectiveness of EMDR (p. 99).

The "all things" episode provides a multisensory experience which, among other things, directs eye movement and gaze, and produces alternating, rhythmic sounds which may stimulate biltateral stimulation. As this author described in the article:

Pulsating chimes, dripping water, ticking clocks and tapping pencils set the rhythm, while slow-motion sequences and extreme close-ups focus viewers' attention. Shots of a window shade toggle undulating back and forth, circulating fans, spinning wheels, flowing curtains, swinging signs and even the main character swaying back and forth while having a mystical experience in a Buddhist temple serve to grasp and direct the gaze of viewers.

(Robertson, 2016, para. 25)

Neurocinematic studies show that the use and positioning of close-ups shots, as exemplified in the episode, influence the modulation of affective and cognitive states, cognitive and narrative processing, and attention and engagement in viewers (Balint & Rooney, 2019; Han et al., 2005). The evocative sequences, extreme close-ups, and slow-motion shots in "all things" may also enhance neural synchrony among viewers. Research has linked neural synchrony to enhanced empathy, social engagement, and cooperation (Lu & Hao, 2019). Neurocinematic studies measure the collective engagement of a group of viewers via their neural synchrony, or intersubject correlation (ISC). Research supports that emotional, evocative film sequences enhance ISC (Lankinen et al., 2014).

Uri Hasson and fellow researchers (2008) are credited with introducing the "new paradigm" of measuring neural synchrony via intersubject correlation to explore "the effects of films on viewer's minds" (p. 21). As Hasson et al. (2008) noted, films are essentially sequences of auditory and visual stimuli which, when meticulously edited into "a coherent whole," can "lead most viewers through a similar sequence of perceptual, emotional and cognitive states ... reflected in the similarity of brain activity (high ISC) across most viewers" (pp. 9–10). These researchers noted that cinematic techniques such as montage, continuity editing, and close-ups have the ability to "direct the viewer's mind during movie watching" and influence their responses.

This author has suggested that increased mindfulness awareness was among the group therapy members' responses while collectively engaged in viewing the "all things" episode. As noted earlier, group members were not only calmer and more reflective immediately after the episode, they were also more communicative and engaged with each other, able to track and describe their experience of the episode, reflect on the personal meaning and significance of the episode, and complete mindfulness exercises focusing on identifying their thoughts, emotions, and sensations. They were essentially demonstrating and reporting core characteristics of mindfulness such as "observing one's moment-to-moment experience, describing one's experiences with words, acting or participating with awareness, and non-judgmental acceptance of one's experiences" (Keng et al., 2011, p. 1045).

Both EMDR and Somatic Experiencing (SE) integrate mindful awareness in their trauma treatment protocols. Vojtová and Hašto (2009) have listed "mindful-like attitude" and somatic awareness among EMDR procedural elements. Similarly, Payne et al. (2015) have noted that SE resembles mindfulness practices which focus on internal awareness (p. 310). According to Siegel (2009), mindfulness awareness has positive effects on brain functioning and "catalyzes the fundamental process of integration" (p. 137).

Mindfulness-based treatments for posttraumatic stress disorder have been effective in targeting core PTSD symptoms, according to Boyd et al. (2018). They reported that recent studies showed that mindfulness-based treatments may help restore connectivity in neural networks such as the DMN in individuals with PTSD. Simon and Engström (2015) have noted that the functioning of the DMN can be used as a biomarker for the therapeutic effects of mindfulness practices. And, as mentioned previously, impaired functioning of the DMN is associated with increased severity of PTSD symptoms, whereas mindfulness practices enhance DMN functioning and are associated with a resting brain state.

Recent neurocinematic research has found that cinema can indeed influence the functioning of the DMN in viewers. Studies conducted by Baldassano et al. (2018) concluded that the functioning of the DMN in individuals viewing cinema "exhibited sequences of activity patterns that were specific to the sequence of events" in the films being viewed (p. 9689). Their findings also showed activation patterns in specific areas of the DMN, notably the mPFC, were "sensitive to overall script structure" and that collective engagement, or ISC, increased as "the script unfolded" (p. 9689).

Cinema and mindfulness practices share another major similarity: both can stimulate empathy. Participating in regular mindfulness practice has been associated with higher levels of empathy in practitioners (Dekeyser et al., 2008). Raz and Hendler (2014) have explored how viewing cinema can influence a somatic form of empathy, referred to as Embodied Simulation, as well as a cognitive form of empathy known as Theory of Mind. Embodied Simulation is activated when an individual experiences an emotional state similar to an individual he/she is observing. This is "emotional mirroring of affective states" according to Raz and Hendler (p. 93). Embodied Simulation is interoceptively driven and is experienced viscerally, whereas Theory of Mind is basically "cognitive perspective-taking." It involves cognitive representations of mental states, as in the ability to ascribe and understand the thoughts, beliefs, motivations, and intentions of another.

Embodied Simulation (ES) and Theory of Mind (ToM) are alternative forms of engagement driven by different neurophysiological systems, and are essentially two different networks which can activate the autonomic nervous system (ANS) in different ways, according to Raz and Hendler (2014). They noted regions in the ES network, which include the ACC and insula, "play a key role in constituting the 'here and now' experiences," whereas the ToM-related network, which includes areas in the mPFC and PFC, is critical in "the retrieval of stored past memories and the anticipations of the future events" (p. 98). Stimulation of the ToM network via cinema can increase or decrease activation of the parasympathetic division of the ANS depending on the characters and content. In contrast, ES network stimulation tends to specifically increase parasympathetic arousal, which is associated with "rest and digest" processes such as decreased muscle tension, decreased heart rate, and relaxation (p. 104).

Raz and Hendler (2014) asserted that neurocinematic research supports the premise that the ES and ToM networks are activated via different cinematic techniques: eso-dramatic and para-dramatic techniques, respectively. Eso-dramatic techniques include "sequences of eyeline-matched shots emphasizing gaze direction" and "combinations of cinematic devices that drive a viewer's engagement based on the somatic and visceral representations ... [and] are perceptual (both auditory and visual)" (p. 104). Para-dramatic techniques include "combinations of cinematic devices that drive a viewer's engagement based on cognitive representations of another's state ... and the alignment of the viewers' and characters' perspectives" (p. 104).

The "all things" episode employs much use of eso-dramatic techniques as exemplified by its extreme close-ups focusing on the eye gaze of the main character, alternating auditory and visual cues, and slow-motion sequences. This may, in part, explain its calming influence on group members as these cinematic techniques activate the ES network, which is associated with corresponding arousal of the parasympathetic nervous system.

Due to its heavy use of eso-dramatic techniques, "all things" has also been useful in introducing clients to basic SE practices and skills, such as the tracking of bodily sensations during scenes which employ these techniques. This author has found that the use of basic SE practices with clients who have PTSD (especially complex PTSD) is most effective and most safely done in individual sessions, however. As noted by van der Kolk (2000), individuals with PTSD are often disconnected from their somatic and emotional states, and traumatic reactions can be triggered when their attention is focused inward. They often are unable to recognize what they are feeling:

> This phenomenon is called "alexithymia," an inability to identify the meaning of physical sensations and muscle activation.... This inability to correctly identify sensations, emotions, and physical states often extends itself to having difficulty appreciating the emotional states and needs of those around them. Unable to gauge and modulate their own internal states they habitually collapse in the face of threat, or lash out in response to minor irritations.
>
> (p. 5)

Van der Kolk (2000) has further noted that the therapeutic treatment of PTSD must allow for clients to "gain distance from their sensory imprints and their traumatic memories so that they can observe and analyze these sensations and emotions without becoming hyperaroused or engaging in avoidance maneuvers" (p. 18). Hyperarousal symptoms such as hypervigilance, sleep disturbance, irritability, difficulty concentrating, and exaggerated startle response are among the most persistent, debilitating and hard to treat symptoms of PTSD (Doron-Lamarca et al., 2015; Schell et al., 2004; van der Kolk, 2000). This author has found severe hyperarousal is particularly prominent in clients with complex PTSD. In children, severe hyperarousal has interfered with their ability to learn coping and self-regulation skills, sustain focus and attention, or become engaged in therapy, much less cinematherapy. Adult clients with severe hyperarousal have similar difficulties and generally cannot tolerate group therapy.

This author has explored the use of a short, animated movie in individual sessions to target hyperarousal symptoms in children and adults who have complex PTSD. The seven-minute movie, entitled *Inscapes*, was selected based on its use of specific neurocinematic techniques which influence DMN functioning and induce a resting brain state while minimizing cognitive and verbal processing. This author wanted to avoid using movies that involved characters or content which could trigger hyperarousal symptoms.

Inscapes was developed by Vanderwal et al. (2015) to be used with children and clinical populations to minimize their distress, improve wakefulness, and avoid the need for sedation while undergoing MRI studies. As the researchers point out, showing movies to healthy adults during neuroimaging studies to facilitate long periods of data collection is common practice. But for children and individuals with mental health disorders—such as PTSD or severe anxiety disorders—who cannot tolerate long periods in MRI scanners and for whom the use of traditional movies may be overstimulating, this practice can make it more difficult to collect the resting brain state data needed for comparison studies.

As Vanderwal et al. (2015) have described it, *Inscapes* is a nonsocial, "low-demand," nonnarrative, animated movie with a soothing musical score. It features slowly moving abstract shapes which flow together without "scene-cuts or camera-based perspective changes" (p. 223). Based on results from their neuroimaging studies, the researchers concluded that this movie "appears to be associated with patterns of FC [functional connectivity] that more closely resemble Rest than those of conventional movies" and the functioning of the default mode network in viewers "did not differ significantly between *Inscapes* and Rest" (p. 231).

This author has used *Inscapes* in individual sessions with 35 clients, ranging in age from 5 years to late 50s, who have complex PTSD and severe hyperarousal symptoms. Clients included 10 males and 15 females

African American/Black, Asian, Caucasian, or Hispanic individuals. Their histories of complex trauma and symptoms of hyperarousal were substantiated via self-report, clinical observation, and scores on ACE, PCL-5, CPSS, and GAD 7 assessments. Client responses were monitored closely for signs of hyperaousal or triggering while they viewed the movie. Clients were asked to describe their experiences as they viewed *Inscapes* or immediately afterward depending on their observed reactions. Clients who appeared to be having significant reactions while viewing the movie were asked to describe their moment-by-moment experiences.

Overall, 23 of 25 clients reported positive, calming experiences while watching *Inscapes*. They were able to maintain focus and attention and describe their experiences while watching the movie and/or immediately after viewing it. Two children under the age of 8, who initially refused to sit down and watch the movie, became actively engaged, focused on viewing the movie and describing their experiences within 90 seconds after the movie was started. Clients who reported positive responses described their experiences as restful, calm, focused, peaceful, and happy. Four adult and two adolescent clients commented specifically on their positive experiences while watching the movie's abstract shapes flowing together and forming new shapes. They identified themes of renewal, transformation, healing, and transcendence while processing their experiences.

One adult and one child reported initial negative and triggering experiences while viewing the movie. The movie was immediately stopped after these clients reported their initial responses, and the clients were then guided through grounding, mindfulness-based exercises and assisted in processing their experience. They reported that they perceived the abstract shapes as shattering, sharp, and confusing.

Inscapes has the potential to be used in individual sessions to help clients with hyperarousal symptoms focus, relax, and practice skills which enhance their ability to identify, express, and process their experiences. It should be used with caution, however. Not all clients will have positive experiences while viewing the movie. The same visual and auditory elements in *Inscapes* which can be soothing to most clients can also be disturbing or triggering to others.

Clinical and Ethical Considerations

When applying neurocinematic research and techniques within trauma therapies and integrative practices, careful consideration must be given to each client's specific treatment needs and goals, trauma history, and potential triggers. These factors must be considered in determining whether the use of cinema is appropriate and in the selection of cinema to be used.

It is essential that therapists be informed about how various cinematic techniques can affect their clients. Factors such as therapeutic rapport and the therapist's knowledge of what forms of cinema their clients enjoy, find meaningful and moving, or disturbing are also crucial. Therapists utilizing neurocinematics in trauma therapies should be well trained and experienced in trauma treatment.

Discussion

Cinema can be both trauma-inducing and therapeutic. Neuroscientists have been using cinema to induce and measure traumatic reactions and symptoms since the 1990s (Nixon et al., 2007; Rauch et al., 1996). While the therapeutic power of cinema has likewise been well documented for decades (Lorusso & Venturini, 2020), the application of neurocinematic research and techniques within psychotherapy is newly emerging. Therefore, the application of neurocinematics within trauma therapies and practices must be managed carefully. When using cinema in the treatment of trauma, Lorusso and Venturini (2020) warn that "care must be taken [lest] the use of film [sets] off environmental triggers thus reactivating traumatic memories" (p. 115).

Neurocinematic research has also shown that specific cinematic techniques can activate and enhance integration in the same areas of the brain and nervous system impaired by traumatic stress, which, as noted by van der Kolk (2006), is needed for effective trauma treatment. When effectively and ethically applied within psychotherapy, neurocinematic research and techniques have the potential to greatly enhance trauma therapies and integrative techniques.

References

Akiki, T., Averill, C., Wrocklage, K., Scott, J., Averill, L., Schwiensburg, B., Alexander-Bloch, A., Martini, B., Southwick, S., Krystal, J., & Abdallah, G. (2018). Default mode network abnormalities in posttraumatic stress disorder: A novel network-restricted topology approach. *Neuroimage, 1*(176), 489–498. doi: 10.1016/j.neuroimage.2018.05.005

Anderson, G. (Writer & director). (2000, April 9). "all things" (Season 7, Episode 17) [Television series episode]. In F. Spotnitz (Executive producer), *The X Files*. Ten Thirteen Productions; 20th Century Fox Television.

Baer, R., Smith, G., Hopkins, J., Krietemeyer, J., & Toney, L. (2006). Using self-report assessment methods to explore facets of mindfulness. *Assessment, 13*, 27–45. doi: 10.1177/1073191105283504

Baldassano, C., Hasson, U., & Norman, K. (2018, November 7). Representation of real-world event schemas during narrative processing. *Journal of Neuroscience, 38*(45), 9689–9699. doi: 10.1523/JNEUROSCI.0251-18.2018

Balint, K., & Rooney, B. (2019). Narrative sequence position of close-ups influences cognitive and affective processing and facilitates theory of mind. *Art and Perception, 7*(1), 27–51. doi: 10.1163/22134913-20191095

Blechert, J., Michael, T., Vriends, N., Margraf, J., & Wilhelm, F. H. (2007). Fear conditioning in posttraumatic stress disorder: Evidence for delayed extinction of autonomic, experiential, and behavioural measures. *Behaviour Research and Therapy*, 45(9), 2019–2033. doi: 10.1016/j.brat.2007.02.012

Boyd, J. E., Lanius, R. A., & McKinnon, M. C. (2018). Mindfulness-based treatments for posttraumatic stress disorder: A review of the treatment literature and neurobiological evidence. *Journal of Psychiatry & Neuroscience*, 43(1), 7–25. doi: 10.1503/jpn.170021

Brown, K., & Ryan, R. (2003). The benefits of being present: Mindfulness and its role in psychological wellbeing. *Journal of Personality and Social Psychology*, 84(4), 822–848. doi: 10.1037/0022-3514.84.4.822

Campbell, K., Shafto, M., Wright, P., Tsvetanov, K., Geerligs, L., & Cusack, R. (2015). Idiosyncratic responding during movie-watching predicted by age differences in attentional control. *Neurobiology of Aging*, 36(11), 3045–3055. doi: 10.1016/j.neurobiolaging.2015.07.028

Cha, H., Chang, W., Shin, D., Jang, D., & Im, C. (2015). EEG-based neurocinematics: Challenges and prospects. *Brain-Computer Interfaces*, 2(4), 186–192. doi: 10.1080/2326263X.2015.1099091

Cohen, J. L., & Johnson, J. L., & Orr, P. P. (Eds.). (2015). *Video and filmmaking as psychotherapy: Research and practice*. Routledge.

Cozolino, L. (2010). *The neuroscience of psychotherapy: Healing the social brain* (2nd ed.). Norton.

Cozolino, L. (2017). *The neuroscience of psychotherapy: Healing the social brain* (3rd ed.). The Norton series on interpersonal neurobiology. Norton.

Dekeyser, M., Raes, F., Leijssen, M., Leysen, S., & Dewulf, D. (2008). Mindfulness skills and interpersonal behaviour. *Personality and Individual Differences*, 44(5), 1235–1245. doi: 10.1016/j.paid.2007.11.018

Doron-LaMarca, S., Niles, B. L., King, D. W., King, L. A., Pless Kaiser, A., & Lyons, M. J. (2015). Temporal associations among chronic PTSD symptoms in U.S. combat veterans. *Journal of Traumatic Stress*, 28(5), 410–417. doi: 10.1002/jts.22039

Han, S., Jiang, Y., Humphreys, G. W., Zhou, T., & Cai, P. (2005). Distinct neural substrates for the perception of real and virtual visual worlds. *Neuroimage*, 24(3), 928–935. doi: 10.1016/j.neuroimage.2004.09.046

Hasson, U., Furman, O., Clark, D., Dudai, Y., & Davachi, L. (2008). Enhanced intersubject correlations during movie viewing correlate with successful episodic encoding. *Neuron*, 57(3), 452–462. doi: 10.1016/j.neuron.2007.12.009

Hasson, U., Nir, Y., Levy, I., Fuhrmann, G., & Malach, R. (2004). Intersubject synchronization of cortical activity during natural vision. *Science*, 303(5664), 1634–1640. doi: 10.1126/science.1089506

Kaltwasser, L., Rost, N., Ardizzi, M., Calbi, M., Settembrino, L., Fingerhut, J., Pauen, M., & Gallese, V. (2019). Sharing the filmic experience – The physiology of socio-emotional processes in the cinema. *PloS ONE*, 14(10), e0223259. doi: 10.1371/journal.pone.0223259

Keng, S.-L., Smoski, M. J., & Robins, C. J. (2011). Effects of mindfulness on psychological health: A review of empirical studies. *Clinical Psychology Review*, 31(6), 1041–1056. doi: 10.1016/j.cpr.2011.04.006

Lankinen, K., Saari, J., Hari, R., & Koskinen, M. (2014). Intersubject consistency of cortical MEG signals during movie viewing. *NeuroImage*, 92, 217–224. doi: 10.1016/j.neuroimage.2014.02.004

Lorusso, L., & Venturini, S. (2020). Cinema and neurology: From history to therapy. In B. Colombo (Ed.), *Brain and art: From aesthetics to therapeutics* (pp. 95–120). Springer. https://link.springer.com/chapter/10.1007/978-3-030-23580-2_9

Lu, K., & Hao, N. (2019). When do we fall in neural synchrony with others? *Social Cognitive and Affective Neuroscience*, 14(3), 253–261. doi: 10.1093/scan/nsz012

Nixon, R. D. V., Nehmy, T., & Seymour, M. (2007). The effect of cognitive load and hyperarousal on negative intrusive memories. *Behaviour Research and Therapy*, 45(11), 2652–2663. doi: 10.1016/j.brat.2007.06.010

Parker, D. B., & Razlighi, Q. R. (2019). Task-evoked negative BOLD response and functional connectivity in the default mode network are representative of two overlapping but separate neurophysiological processes. *Scientific Reports*, 9(1), 14473. doi: 10.1038/s41598-019-50483-8

Payne, P., Levine, P. A., & Crane-Godreau, M. A. (2015). Somatic experiencing: Using interoception and proprioception as core elements of trauma therapy. *Frontiers in Psychology*, 6, 93. doi: 10.3389/fpsyg.2015.00093

Rauch, S. L., van der Kolk, B. A., Fisler, R. E., Alpert, N. M., Orr, S. P., Savage, C. R., Fischman, A. J., Jenike, M. A., & Pittman, R. K. (1996). A symptom provocation study of posttraumatic stress disorder using positron emission tomography and script-driven imagery. *Archives of General Psychiatry*, 53(5), 380–387. doi: 10.1001/archpsyc.1996.01830050014003

Raz, G., & Hendler, T. (2014). Forking cinematic paths to the self: Neurocinematically informed model of empathy in motion pictures. *Projections*, 8(2), 89–114. doi: 10.3167/proj.2014.080206

Robertson, B. (2016, March 29). All things connect: The integration of mindfulness, cinema, and psychotherapy. *Counseling Today*. https://ct.counseling. org/2016/03/all-things-connect-the-integration-of-mindfulness-cinema-and-psychotherapy/#

Rombold-Bruehl, F., Otte, C., Renneberg, B., Hellmann-Regen, J., Bruch, L., Wingenfeld, K., & Roepke, S. (2018, December). Impact of stress response systems on forced choice recognition in an experimental trauma film paradigm. *Neurobiology of Learning and Memory*, 156, 45–52. doi: 10.1016/j.nlm.2018.10.010

Schell, T. L., Marshall, G. N., & Jaycox, L. H. (2004). All symptoms are not created equal: The prominent role of hyperarousal in the natural course of posttraumatic psychological distress. *Journal of Abnormal Psychology*, 113(2), 189–197. doi: 10.1037/0021-843X.113.2.189

Schultebraucks, K., Rombold-Bruehl, F., Wingenfeld, K., Hellman-Regen, J., Otte, C. & Roepke, S. (2019, July 8). Heightened biological stress response during exposure to trauma film predicts an increase in intrusive memories. *Journal of Abnormal Psychology*, 128(7), 645–657. doi: 10.1037/abn0000440

Sherin, J. E., & Nemeroff, C. B. (2011). Post-traumatic stress disorder: The neurobiological impact of psychological trauma. *Dialogues in Clinical Neuroscience*, 13(3), 263–278. doi: 10.31887/dcns.2011.13.1/jsherin

Siegel, D. J. (2009). Mindful awareness, mindsight, and neural integration. *The Humanistic Psychologist*, 37(2), 137–158. doi: 10.1080/08873260902892220

Siegel, D. J. (2010). *Mindsight: The new science of personal transformation*. Bantam Books.

Simon, R., & Engström, M. (2015, June 9). The default mode network as a bio-marker for monitoring the therapeutic effects of meditation. *Frontiers in Psychology, 6,* 776. doi: 10.3389/fpsyg.2015.00776

Sonkusare, S., Breakspear, M., & Guo, C. (2019). Naturalistic stimuli in neurosci-ence: Critically acclaimed. *Trends in Cognitive Sciences, 23*(8), 699–714. doi: 10.1016/j.tics.2019.05.004

Uhlhaas, P., & Singer, W. (2006). Neural synchrony in brain disorders: Relevance for cognitive dysfunctions and pathophysiology. *Neuron, 52*(1), 155–168. doi: 10.1016/j.neuron.2006.09.020

van der Kolk, B. (2000). Posttraumatic stress disorder and the nature of trauma. *Dialogues in Clinical Neuroscience, 2*(1), 7–22. doi: 10.31887/DCNS.2000.2.1/ bvdkolk

van der Kolk, B. (2004). Psychobiology of posttraumatic stress disorder. *Textbook of biological psychiatry.* Wiley Online Library.

van der Kolk, B. (2005). Developmental trauma disorder: Toward a rational diag-nosis for children with complex trauma histories. *Psychiatric Annals, 35*(5), 401–408. doi: 10.3928/00485713-20050501-06

van der Kolk, B. (2006, August). Clinical implications of neuroscience research in PTSD. *Annals of the New York Academy of Sciences, 1071*(1), 277–293. doi: 10.1196/annals.1364.022

Vanderwal, T., Kelly, C., Eilbott, J., Mayes, L. C., & Castellanos, F. X. (2015). Inscapes: A movie paradigm to improve compliance in functional magnetic resonance imaging. *NeuroImage, 122,* 222–232. doi: 10.1016/j. neuroimage.2015.07.069

Viard, A., Mutlu, J., Chanraud, S., Guénolé, F., Egler, P.-J., Gérardin, P., Baleyte, J., Dayan, J., Eustache, F., & Guillery-Girard, B. (2019). Altered default mode network connectivity in adolescents with post-traumatic stress disorder. *NeuroImage: Clinical, 22,* 101731. doi: 10.1016/j.nicl.2019.101731

Vojtová, H., & Hašto, J. (2009). Neurobiology of eye movement desensitization and reprocessing. *Activitas Nervosa Superior, 51*(3), 98–102. doi: 10.1007/ BF03379925

Welton, R., & Kay, J. (2015, October 22). The neurobiology of psychotherapy. *PsychiatricTimes,32*(10).https://www.psychiatrictimes.com/view/neurobiology-psychotherapy

4 Creating Videogames for Psychotherapy

Christopher R. Harz

Introduction

The therapeutic effect of creating art in traditional visual media such as painting and sculpture has a history of many centuries (Malchiodi, 2007). Celebrated leaders famously stated that painting helped them relax and refresh. For instance, Winston Churchill created over 500 paintings, which he claimed "saved his sanity" and helped him overcome the "black dog" of severe depression (Churchill, 1948). Interestingly, Churchill found that paintings where he had inserted himself in the scene were especially effective. Such art therapy was formalized in the U.S. by Margaret Naumburg, Edith Kramer, and others (Rubin, 1988).

The discovery of therapeutic effects from the creation of films and videos is more recent, and coincided in large part both with the availability of inexpensive and easy-to-use video creation and editing tools and recent scientific research into the effectiveness of such creation by therapists such as Cohen, Chin, and others (Chin et al., 1980; Cohen et al., 2015; Furman, 1990; Gardano, 1994, etc.). Research into therapeutic effects of film creation, especially by amateurs, was not limited to specific purposes such as trauma reduction but also included increasing social skills, improving feelings of self-worth and accomplishment, and relieving stress and depression (Cohen).

An interesting course of intervention has been the creation and implementation by therapist teachers of intensive, short "boot camp" instructional classes for patients in the creation of films and videos, including storyboarding, filming, acting, directing, and editing (Tuval-Mashiach & Patton, 2015; Tuval-Mashiach et al., 2018). A more recent development is the therapist-led creation of videogames by patients. Videogames created by professional game companies have been used for psychotherapy for over two decades. One famous example is the creation of *Virtual Iraq* by USC's Institute for Creative Technologies (ICT), which has been shown to be highly effective in treating military PTSD patients (Rizzo et al., 2004). Such therapeutic games were typically administered by trained therapists, with only limited input from patients. A major block was the

DOI: 10.4324/9781315622507-6

complexity and expense of videogames. In the 1980s, programming easily ran into millions of dollars and needed large teams of professionals, and graphics boards and headsets could cost over $100,000 each.

Recent advances in software such as the ability to create games with easy-to-use programs such as JavaScript and HTML5 and game engines such as Unity, as well as the availability of low-cost (below $100) graphics processing units (GPUs) and head-mounted displays (HMDs) such as the Oculus Rift ($600–$1,500), now make it possible for amateurs to participate in the creation or modification of videogames, both as a therapeutic exercise per se and in partnership with therapy-related game creators, to make such games more effective and immersive. This chapter addresses this topic.

The Potential for Videogame-Based Psychotherapy

Videogame-based therapy, like other means of therapeutic intervention, should of course be administered by professionals, to assure that ethical guidelines are met and to monitor and measure effectiveness and outcomes. With such careful management by mental health professionals, videogames could offer potential advantages for therapies involving art creation, including the following:

1   With modern tools, videogames can be easier to create or modify than traditional visual arts such as painting, which can take many months to master, and appear unsuited for interventions such as short, intensive "boot camp" courses to teach game creation or modification.

2   The interactive nature of videogames can increase involvement and motivation. As an example, it has been demonstrated that a pain diversion game such as BreakAway's *Free Dive*, which is designed for pain reduction for children undergoing chemotherapy and other painful treatments, is several times as effective if the patient can interact with a graphical user interface (GUI) to navigate through the game world, rather than merely passively watch the attractive underwater scenery (HCP*Live*, 2010).

3   Realistic or fantasy game worlds can offer an increased scope of self-expression that might be more difficult to create with filmic production. Although much virtual content is possible with movies via green screens, such worlds can be easier to create in a game, especially for low-budget or amateur productions (Ehinger, 2015).

4   Videogames do not need to be created from scratch, unlike many film or video productions. Game producers can take advantage of existing worlds, libraries of 3D animated characters, and so on. Some of this is possible with film, which allows insertion of photographs from stock libraries, for instance, but this is much more limited. One

example of this is machinima, where an individual or team can enter an existing game world such as *Second Life* as avatars, act out a story, and capture the complete sequence of action, all without the need for actual ("practical") sets or props (Lowood, 2008; Thomas, 2017).

5   Games can use biofeedback from wearable and other sensors, so that body-state indicators, including emotion tracking, can be incorporated into the game.

6   Games can feature a choice of intensity and paths, with "leveling." Existing game engines support the creation of different levels (game areas) for higher or lower intensity and skill levels. It is somewhat possible to do this with multitrack films with different outcomes and endings, but that is more limited and difficult.

7   Videogames can involve worlds with nonhuman characters, to circumvent religious or cultural taboos. For example, a film where a female touches a man would be taboo in Saudi Arabia, and characters of different races might stir controversy in some countries, but nonrealistic characters such as those easily created in *Second Life* may avoid such controversy. Films can use puppets or animation for a similar effect, but this can be much more difficult.

8   Creating movies and videos is highly attractive, with many modern filmmakers such as Spielberg and Lucas becoming folk heroes. Videogames, however, have an extra "coolness" factor, with over 90 percent of Americans playing them. Therapy with videogames has been shown to have much higher retention rates than traditional therapies, especially for males in military or law enforcement (Rizzo et al., 2021).

9   New virtual reality (VR) technology such as Oculus Rift headsets offer high levels of immersion in 3D virtual worlds. Filmic production of VR is also possible, with 360-degree cameras, but such worlds are two-dimensional and are difficult to make interactive.

10 VR videogame creation also offers the possibility of "dual purpose" therapy: that is, the creation of therapist-led intensive classes that teach patients VR skills that not only have therapeutic outcomes but could also lead to job skills. Whereas there is a limited market for short-form movies, the market for short-form (ten minutes or less) VR content is rapidly increasing, as is major investment in this area. Dual-purpose classes may be much easier to fund for groups such as military veterans, since it may be easier to demonstrate an ROI for the graduates: in addition to therapeutic benefits, they could then use their new skills to find jobs in the intensely dynamic international VR market.

Videogame Creation Methods

This section explores different methods that therapists can use to enable patients to create user-generated content (UGC, or "user-gen") for videogames, including games intended to have therapeutic effects for an individual patient and games that can be shared with communities of health professionals for a larger audience. User-generated content is not new. Many games such as *Little Big Planet, Minecraft, Trials Evolution, The Sims 2*, and *Team Fortress 2* have supported extensive input from users, including the provision of "building brick" objects in the game to create buildings, farms, and military formations. Players have also modified or "modded" many games. Such UGC was either limited in scope or involved professional programming skills and was generally not useful for easy storytelling or self-expression. New technology can enable amateurs (such as therapy patients) to explore new vistas of UGC, including using it for storytelling and modifying or even creating VR worlds. Motivation for such user-gen could include guidance by the therapist, the "fun factor" of creating something, recognition or awards for skilled creations, and the ability to share such content with others. Methods that can be used by therapists to guide UGC by their patients/users include the following:

- **Personalization of existing videogames.** The more a player relates to his or her avatar in the game, the more immersive the experience tends to be. Putting a user's face onto an avatar used to be a professional, expensive project. However, as was demonstrated at the 2016 Game Developers Conference, new software such as Uraniom and itSeez3D enable a player to have his or her face captured via a panoramic videotape by an HP tablet or other devices, and—in less than a minute—that face can be inserted onto a game avatar. From then on, the user sees not a generic figure in the virtual world, but one with his or her face. New versions of the software can do a full-body scan, and a 3D "action figure" can then be produced locally by a 3D printer.

- **Sandbox creation of virtual worlds.** Existing or new videogames can now incorporate an area (a "sandbox") with tools that enable the user to easily create objects for a world, including buildings, streets, monsters, puzzles, etc. An added feature is voice or typed recording of the user as they explain what is being created or added to the game world, and why. The level of creation can range from moving virtual objects around to creating custom maps of areas to play in. The popularity of such user-gen is demonstrated by the popularity of *The Sims*, a building game that is one of the most popular videogames ever created.

- **Purchase of virtual objects.** Worlds such as *Second Life* enable users to cheaply purchase a wide range of fantasy objects, including clothing or costumes, customized avatars (e.g., an avatar that looks like an animal), motions (e.g., dance moves for music), and living spaces. The range and number of such objects can assure that no two players will look or act the same.

- **Creation of characters.** In addition to the creation and live movement of their own avatar in a game world, a user can also create other characters (NPCs, or non-player characters) with customized motivations, looks, and behaviors. Character creation "from scratch" is still difficult, but drop-down menus of a wide range of choices can enable a user to populate a game with AI-driven figures representing parents, school bullies, enemies, lovers, and friends.
- **Machinima.** A single user or team of players can enter a game area via their avatars and act out a play or scenario. All actions can be captured (from different points of view) and replayed later, to give the user a "third person" perspective of actions and behavior patterns.

Therapeutic Applications for Videogames with User-Generated Content

A sample (not comprehensive) list of potential interventions using videogames includes the following:

- **Post-traumatic stress disorder.** PTSD is a major problem in the U.S., with over 300,000 veterans evidencing clinical levels of it, requiring new levels of therapeutic effectiveness (Yehuda et al., 2015). Symptoms include intrusive recollections, emotional numbing, and hyperarousal by incidents (such as loud noises) reminiscent of the combat theater. Videogames such as *Virtual Iraq* which enable exposure therapy have shown great effectiveness in reducing PTSD (Rizzo et al., 2009). Other PTSD games include *Virtual Vietnam, World Trade Center*, and *Terrorist Bus Bombing*. Users could generate additional content to make such therapy games even more relevant and effective. Users have already had an active role in contributing to *Virtual Iraq*, according to Rizzo et al. (2004), who said that the relative lack of terrain features and objects in the game was a positive feature, as patients used their imaginations to fill in details. Videogames such as *Virtual Iraq* are also great examples of how therapy games can reuse the digital assets of existing games; *Virtual Iraq* was built on top of *Full Spectrum Warrior*, a popular game for the Xbox.
- **Phobias and anxiety disorders.** A number of videogames exist for phobias such as fear of flying or claustrophobia, involving the use of VR for exposure therapy (Botella et al., 1998; Parsons & Rizzo, 2008; Powers & Emmelkamp, 2008). However, experience has shown that "one size fits all" game worlds may not be optimal, and that user input and some customization of the virtual sets could make the therapy more immersive (Wiederhold & Bouchard, 2014).

- **Drug addiction.** Addictions to drugs, gambling, and other repetitive stimulations tend to involve a failure to recognize patterns and denial of likely consequences of a behavior pattern. The U.S. military has pioneered the use of VR for mission rehearsal exercises (MRXs) for training. MRXs involve proceeding through a set of behaviors (a "mission") in a virtual world (e.g., with networked tank simulators) and exploring options and their consequences before going into the actual mission (e.g., armored combat with an Iraqi tank battalion) (Hill et al., 2003). Similar procedures are being tried with VR games that can enable an addict to recognize repetitive behavior patterns, identify addictive stimuli (such as interaction with enablers), and experience likely consequences.

- **Performance improvement.** The U.S. Air Force's Human Research Laboratory, DARPA (Defense Advanced Research Projects Agency), and other military R&D agencies have been using videogames to exploit novel brain-computer interfaces (BCIs) to improve human performance by reducing unwanted stress while increasing positive stimulation, using wearable devices. A major aspect of this research was the analysis of Narrative Networks (N2) and the powerful influence they have on human thoughts, emotions, and behavior (Casebeer & Russell, 2005). A second research avenue has been using VR to help restore neural and behavioral functions of soldiers disabled by combat or accidents (Miranda et al., 2015). The potential exists for extending existing prototypes produced from these research efforts into usable products for the general public, with user-generated inputs to turn generalized procedures into specific therapeutic applications.

References

Botella, C., Baños, R. M., Perpiñá, C., Villa, H., Alcañiz, M., & Rey, A. (1998). Virtual reality treatment of claustrophobia: A case report. *Behaviour Research and Therapy, 36*(2), 239–246. doi: 10.1016/s0005-7967(97)10006-7

Casebeer, W. D., & Russell, J. A. (2005, March). Storytelling and terrorism: Towards a comprehensive "counter-narrative strategy". *Strategic Insights, 4*(3). http://citeseerx.ist.psu.edu/viewdoc/download?doi=10.1.1.116.7615&rep=rep1&type=pdf

Chin, R. J., Chin, M. M., Palombo, P., Palombo, C., Bannasch, G., & Cross, P. M. (1980). Project Reachout: Building social skills through art and video. *The Arts in Psychotherapy, 7*(4), 281–284. doi: 10.1016/0197-4556(80)90007-6

Churchill, W. S. (1948). *Painting as a pastime*. Oldhams Press.

Cohen, J. L. Johnson, J. L., & Orr, P. P. (Eds.). (2015). *Video and filmmaking as psychotherapy: Research and practice*. Routledge.

Ehinger, J. (2015). Filming the fantasy: Green screen technology from novelty to psychotherapy. In J. L. Cohen, J. L. Johnson, & P. P. Orr (Eds.), *Video and filmmaking as psychotherapy: Research and practice* (pp. 43–54). Routledge.

Furman, L. (1990). Video therapy: An alternative for the treatment of adolescents. *The Arts in Psychotherapy, 17,* 165–169. doi: 10.1016/0197-4556(90)90027-N

Gardano, A. (1994). Creative video therapy with early adolescent girls in short-term treatment. *Journal of Child & Adolescent Group Therapy, 4*(2), 99–116. doi: 10.1007/BF02548483

HCP*Live.* (2010, May 7). Virtual reality offers exciting possibilities for pain management. https://www.hcplive.com/view/virtual_reality_pain_management

Hill, R. W., Gratch, J., Marsella, S., Rickel, J., Swartout, W., & Traum, D. R. (2003). Virtual humans in the Mission Rehearsal Exercise system. *Künstliche Intelligenz, 17,* 5–10.

Lowood, H. (2008). Found technology: Players as innovators in the making of machinima. In T. McPherson (Ed.), *Digital youth, innovation, and the unexpected* (pp. 165–196). MIT Press. doi: 10.1162/dmal.9780262633598.165

Malchiodi, C. A. (2007). *The art therapy sourcebook.* McGraw-Hill.

Miranda, R. A., Casebeer, W. D., Hein, A. M., Judy, J. W., Krotkov, E. P., Laabs, T. L., Manzo, J. E., Pankratz, K. G., Pratt, G. A., Sanchez, J. C., Weber, D. J., Wheeler, T. L., & Ling, G. S. F. (2015, April 9). DARPA-funded efforts in the development of novel brain-computer interface technologies. *Journal of Neuroscience Methods, 244,* 52–67. doi: 10.1016/j.jneumeth.2014.07.019

Parsons, T. D., & Rizzo, A. A. (2008). Affective outcomes of virtual reality exposure therapy for anxiety and specific phobias: A meta-analysis. *Journal of Behavioural Therapy and Experimental Psychiatry, 39,* 250–261. doi: 10.1016/j.jbtep.2007.07.007

Powers, M. B., & Emmelkamp, P. M. G. (2008). Virtual reality exposure therapy for anxiety disorders: A meta-analysis. *Journal of Anxiety Disorders, 22,* 561–569. doi: 10.1016/j.janxdis.2007.04.006

Rizzo, A., Hartholt, A., & Mozgai, S. (2021). Establishment of clinical virtual reality: Methodologies from the front lines of Afghanistan to COVID-19. In W. Greenleaf, L. Roberts, & R. Fine (Eds.), *Applied virtual reality in healthcare: Case studies and perspectives* (pp. 163–188). Cool Blue Media.

Rizzo, A., Reger, G., Gahm, G., Difede, J. A., & Rothbaum, B. O. (2009). Virtual reality exposure therapy for combat-related PTSD. In P. J. Shiromani, T. M. Keane, & J. E. LeDoux (Eds.), *Post-Traumatic Stress Disorder: Basic science and clinical practice* (pp. 375–399). Humana Press.

Rizzo, A. A., Pair, J., McNerney, P. J., Eastlund, E., Manson, B., Gratch, J., Hill, R., Swartout, B., & Roy, M. (2004). *An immersive virtual reality therapy application for Iraq War veterans with PTSD: From training to toy to treatment.* University of Southern California, Institute for Creative Technologies. https://www.researchgate.net/publication/235064931_An_Immersive_Virtual_Reality_Therapy_Application_for_Iraq_War_Veterans_with_PTSD_From_Training_to_Toy_to_Treatment

Rubin, J. A. (1988). Art counseling: An alternative. *Elementary School Guidance & Counseling, 22*(3), 180–185. http://www.jstor.org/stable/42868819

Thomas, K. (2017). IBM Watson AI XPRIZE. Kelland Thomas. Retrieved January 29, 2022, from http://www.kellandthomas.com/projects.html

Tuval-Mashiach, R., & Patton, B. (2015). Digital storytelling: Healing for the YouTube generation of veterans. In J. L. Cohen, J. L. Johnson, & P. P. Orr (Eds.), *Video and filmmaking as psychotherapy: Research and practice* (pp. 146–162). Routledge.

Tuval-Mashiach, R., Patton, B. W., & Drebing, C. (2018). "When you make a movie, and you see your story there, you can hold it": Qualitative exploration of collaborative filmmaking as a therapeutic tool for veterans. *Frontiers in Psychology*, *9*, 1954. doi: 10.3389/fpsyg.2018.01954

Wiederhold, B. K., & Bouchard, S. (2014). *Advances in virtual reality and anxiety disorders*. Springer.

Yehuda, R., Hoge, C. W., McFarlane, A. C., Vermetten, E., Lanius, R. A., Nievergelt, C. M., Hobfoll, S. E., Koenen, K. C., Neylan, T. C., & Hyman, S. E. (2015). Post-traumatic stress disorder. *Nature Reviews Disease Primers*, *1*(1). doi: 10.1038/nrdp.2015.57. Note: Bookmark and reformat this listing.

5 My Journey through Breast Cancer[1]

Penelope P. Orr

Introduction

My journey started with my best friend mentioning to me that she was going to get a mammogram because, in the doctor's office in which she works, she had seen a large number of women come through who had recently been diagnosed with breast cancer. As my friend was talking, I realized that I had skipped my last two mammograms because I was too busy, and I didn't think that I was likely to get breast cancer. I had breastfed two children, and my family had no history of breast cancer. However, when my friend mentioned that she was going to get her mammogram, I thought I should probably do so as well. That was January of 2014. I soon received a phone call from my doctor saying that they had found an "abnormality" in my mammogram and that they would like me to come back to get a diagnostic mammogram.

Starting My Digital Journal

The previous August, I had applied for a Fulbright scholar award to work with expressive therapists at the University of Roehampton to develop a digital journaling method that could be used across the expressive therapies. I had also finished helping Dr. Cohen and Dr. Johnson (Cohen et al., 2015) in editing a book on the use of video and film in psychotherapy. These ideas came together with my research on Ira Progoff's journaling method (Progoff, 1992). Since I had been mulling in my head over these projects and ideas, I decided, upon learning that I might have breast cancer, that I would use a digital journaling process to help me with the stress of this illness. I could both learn and experience personally this process that I was researching while, at the same time, taking care of my mental health.

Progoff (1992) stated that journaling "enables us to draw our lives into focus at a given moment amid pressures of a crisis so that we can resolve immediate issues" (p. 7). The collection of immediate feelings and thoughts were to be written in the daily journal. At a later time, those immediate thoughts and emotions would be reexamined, metaphors were to be

DOI: 10.4324/9781315622507-7

developed, and depth reflection would be possible through other sections of the Progoff journal method, such as speaking with your inner wisdom. To put these ideas into a digital video journal as I had planned, I decided just to record items throughout my days, and save them in files as my daily journal. But then I moved from an "abnormality" in my breast to a BRCA 4C assessment by the radiologist (which meant that it was 80% likely that it was cancer). After my ultrasound, I realized that merely recording my days with the cell phone was not going to be much help in dealing with my feelings. So I started to create visual journal entries to express the emotions that came with my diagnosis, as well as recording audio and video and taking still pictures. I found that the video captures documented my process, and helped me to remember what I needed to remember since mentally I was feeling overwhelmed. The visual artistic entries in my journal helped me to express my immediate emotions so that I could refocus on my family and daily life while I waited for more information.

While in the diagnostic stage of my treatment, I was too worried about what might happen, how it would affect my family, my job, and my life to do more than capture images and express direct feelings. I was not ready for Progoff's (1992) Stepping Stones exercises. The Stepping Stones enable the journaler "to draw out the jumbled mass of life experiences; the thin threads that carry our potentialities through their phases of development toward a fuller unfolding" (76). I could only see negative potentialities and was not ready to look more deeply.

After my biopsy, I was officially diagnosed with invasive lobular cancer. Once I had the official diagnosis, prognosis, and next steps in my treatment, my mind calmed down a great deal, and I was able to begin reflecting on the images that I had created or collected up to that point. I sat down and reviewed all the video footage, pictures, and artwork that I had created to that point. By studying the images I had collected, I realized two things. I realized that I spent a lot of time on the road traveling to and from doctor's appointments, and I seemed to use that time to process what I had learned so that I could be healthy at home for my husband and son. I also found that my healthy life continued right next to my stressed "cancer" life. My son still had his birthday; we always vacationed in South Carolina, and I even enjoyed sightseeing with my family. Life went on while I was dealing with my shock, but capturing the images and knowing that I would come back to them later to analyze them allowed me to set aside my stress so that I could be in the joy of the moment with my family. For me, that was probably one of the most beneficial aspects of the digital journaling process at this point.

Refining My Digital Journal Process

As I progressed from diagnosis to double mastectomy to recovery, I continued the multimedia aspect of my digital journal by expressing my feelings through visual journaling and capturing the process with my phone camera. My sister came up from South Carolina to care for me during my surgery. When my sister came up, and I prepared to go into the hospital, I actually planned on videotaping the experience. I even packed my journal and art materials to take to the hospital; however, once I was checked in and right through until I left, I did not record anything. No pictures; no art-making; no video was taken at the hospital. It took planning and forethought and energy to do those things, and while at the hospital, I found I just didn't have it in me. I was in survival mode (Figures 5.1 and 5.2).

The outpouring of concern from family and friends that was shown to me seemed to refill me after I had been emptied. This happened while in the hospital and upon my arrival home. The flowers, cards, emails, visits, and food that was showered upon me filled me with hope, and with the realization that a lot of people cared about me. Something about being a caregiver, as I have always been in my profession and home life, made me forget that I also need others to care for me. I used this care as a starting point for getting back to being able to journal, and to reflect and heal.

My journaling process had an established pattern to it at this point in its collection process, and mentally I was continuing to mull over what I was creating but was not yet ready to work beyond the visual to put my thoughts into words or an organized structure. It wasn't until after I had finished with my physical therapy that I was able to take the next step in the journaling process: making meaning. At that point, my wounds were simply red lines across my chest, and my oncologist declared me free of cancer.

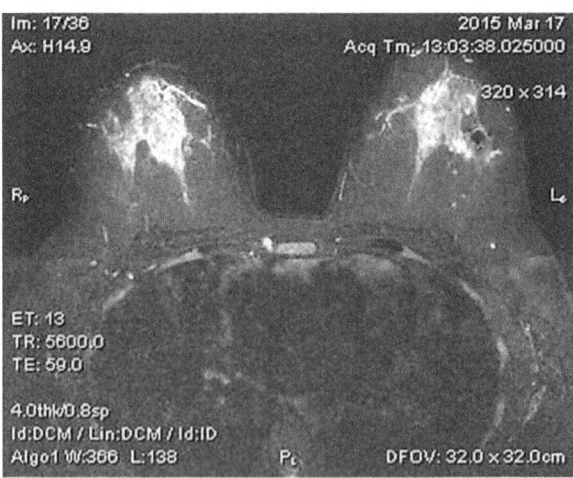

Figure 5.1 MRI showing the cancer.

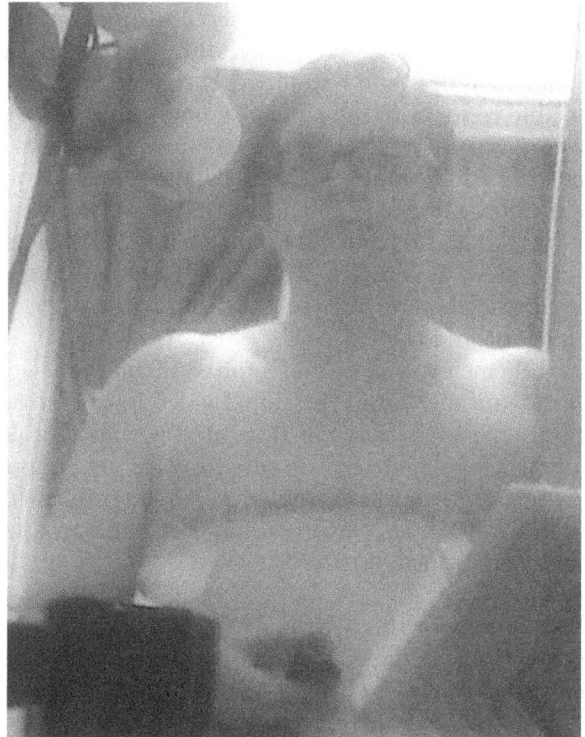

Figure 5.2 After double mastectomy.

As Progoff (1992) wrote:

> The first step is to acknowledge the problems of our life as we find
> them, to observe them and describe them as objectively as we can.
> That gives us a reference point in outer reality, but we do not estab-
> lish our position there. We drawback. We move away from the sur-
> face of things. We move inward in order to return with a greater
> resource to use in re-approaching the situation.... The atmosphere of
> inward attention seems to possess a profound validity that dwarfs
> any particular opinions, or any particular anxieties we may hold
> about the details of our existence.
>
> (p. 9)

Going Deeper

I had acknowledged a specific problem of my life, observed it, and
described it through video. The problem gave me a reference point in my
outer reality to establish where I was, and to be able to draw back. It was

in the editing process of the images gathered throughout my breast cancer experience that I was able to move inward to find validity in my experience and to understand the impact this experience had on my persona. I was able to identify the emotions involved in those experiences. Through the movement of images, the juxtaposing of them, the overlapping of them, the addition of sound, and playing freely with the element of time, I was able to find new and additional reactions that I wasn't able to sense at the time. I asked questions such as "What emotions and awareness are stirred in you?" (p. 210), and "Do you feel in its symbolism a particular theme or thread?" (p. 210), plus others posed by Progoff (1992), to help me find more depth.

The central theme or symbol that I found through the editing process was that of the journey. I built the edited video journal around this concept. The journey—or, as Campbell termed it, the "hero's journey"—stems from archetypal imagery, as put forward by Jung (1949/1993). Archetypes are patterns of behaviors or symbolic imagery present in the minds of all individuals. They express significant human concerns such as birth, death, love, survival, family, etc.

> [T]he first works of the hero is to retreat from the world scene of secondary effects to those causal zones of the psyche where the difficulties really reside, and there to clarify the difficulties, eradicate them in his own case [...] and breakthrough to the undistorted, direct experience and assimilation of what C. G. Jung has called "the archetypal images." [...] The archetypes to be discovered and assimilated are precisely those that have inspired, throughout the annals of human culture, the basic images of ritual, mythology, and vision.
>
> (Campbell, 1949/1993, pp. 17–20)

The specific hero's journey that I think I found in the editing process of my journal is *the quest to rid the land of danger* (Volger, 2007). As Volger's stages of the journey indicate, my own journal starts by showing my everyday life; then, I was called to adventure by the possibility of breast cancer. I didn't want to start on my journey to overcoming cancer, but I had no choice. I was then mentored by wonderful nurses, doctors, and other cancer survivors. I met allies along the way and fought my enemy at different stages. The surgery itself was the ordeal I faced in the innermost cave, in which no one was allowed but me. I was rewarded for surviving death by the outpouring of care from my family and friends, and I found a road back to my ordinary life. The "elixir" that I took away from this journey was learning that caretakers sometimes need others to care for them. I was not a traditional "hero" in the sense that I was willing to sacrifice my own needs for others, but I was ready to go through trials to get healthy so that I could continue to take care of my family. Cancer itself acted like a shape-shifter as I learned something new about it with each test, and it grew and changed during the time of testing. My allies and mentors were my family, my nursing caregivers, and my doctors. I think the trickster came into play early in the diagnostic process, when I would go through periods of thinking that it wasn't going to be cancer that I faced. I was not conscious of how well the editing of my journal fits the hero's journey, as Campbell described it, until I finished work on the editing and started writing this chapter.

Concerns

While working on this project and working through my cancer, I had some concerns. An incident happened while I was in the editing process. After I had been editing the video aspect of the journal for several days, I had a vivid dream in which I found myself on an operating table, and the doctor and nurse were inserting tubes into my lungs. The insertion of the first tube caused me to choke and cough up blood, and when they inserted the second tube, the choking stopped. I did not feel pain, but I couldn't move, and I was horrified when the doctors took off their gloves and prepared to leave. I understood in the dream that the tubes were a prep procedure and that the surgery was scheduled for the next morning. I also knew that they were going to leave me like that all night.

I woke up flat on my back in bed with all my muscles rigid, and I was shaking uncontrollably. I believe that in my review of the video, delving into the emotional aspects of the cancer journey had reawakened my muscle memory from the time I was under anesthesia during surgery. So, my concern for others doing a similar journaling process after a medical procedure is that this visual review of trauma may retraumatize the journaler, or bring to the surface trauma that might have been buried. I think that physical memory was missing from my journal, and needed to come to the surface for me to process it, but I was not expecting it. Thus, it is essential that this process, if undertaken with a specific trauma in mind, be done under a therapist's supervision, and that the therapy continues after the journaling is done.

Another concern I had throughout the filming of the items for my journal was the concept of privacy. There were many instances when I filmed in public spaces, in which there was no expectation of privacy, such as during the spa day near the end of my journaling process. The spa day was a public event for cancer patients. The local TV news was even there, covering the event. Also, though I had no obligation to protect the privacy of the other attendees who had cancer, I didn't want to do any harm by showing their faces when they might not be aware that I was filming. My level of comfort in filming dictated that I not exhibit faces of those I interacted within the process of my cancer treatment. The only people I fully share are my family, as they all approved me, putting them in the film. A discussion with a therapist about privacy, legal as well as felt, needs to occur with a client making a multimedia digital journal. The therapist needs to know the confidentiality and privacy codes in the Art Therapy Credentials Board code of professional practice if the client ever chooses to show their journal to others.

Overall, this process of collecting my journal items kept me sane during a stressful time in my life. The editing process helped me to reevaluate my feelings during that process, find new depths that I was not able to approach during the cancer treatment, and find closure for my experience. I feel like I have created something in my final film version of the journal that will help my family understand what I went through, as well as helping others to understand the process and feelings associated with a breast cancer diagnosis. I also learned what worked for me individually in the digital journaling process, and this knowledge will help me move my research forward, teach other expressive therapists, and work with my current and future clients. I am now back where I started on this journey: looking forward to researching with expressive therapists in the UK to further develop a digital journaling process; spending time with my family; making my art; and teaching. Life is good.

Note

1 Author's note: This research was partially made possible by a Fulbright Scholar Award. The opinions and ideas of this chapter are solely those of the author and do not reflect those of the Fulbright Foundation.

References

Campbell, J. (1993). *The hero with a thousand faces*. Fontana Press. (Original work published 1949)

Cohen, J. L., Johnson, J. L., & Orr, P. P. (Eds.) (2015). Video and filmmaking *as psychotherapy: Research and practice*. Routledge.

Progoff, I. (1992). *At a journal workshop: Writing to access the power of the unconscious and evoke creative ability*. Penguin Putnam.

Volger, C. (2007). *The writer's journey: Mythic structures for writers*. Michael Wiese Productions.

Part III
Trauma in the United States

6 Process Language and Its Impact

Making a Digital Cancer Narrative with Adolescent and Young Adult Cancer Patients and Survivors

Lila Pereira, Kimberly Marynowski and Katie DiCola

Introduction

Adolescent and young adult (AYA) oncology patients experience a significant burden of their cancer experience not typically seen in patients younger or older. This is largely due to the disruption in normal maturation during a key time of identity development when coping skills are typically learned and patients cultivate a higher level of insight into their illness compared to younger patients. Due to logistical and illness-related barriers (e.g., isolation, lack of access to mental health staff, and inability to talk to same-aged peers), patients may seek other ways to process their illness experience. While previous generations have utilized expressive writing, recent literature has suggested that the current generation of AYA patients (millennials and gen Z) prefer high-tech methods of expression, including video and film. The current study examined the usage of video testimonials, similar to those seen on YouTube, in a group of AYA cancer patients and survivors (diagnosed between ages 15 and 39) to identify how video may allow patients to process their cancer experiences and reap personal benefits from making the film. Results suggested that in the second half of the film, when AYAs were able to spend more time talking about themselves, they often utilized processing-based language and saw positive results from discussing their cancer experience on film. This adds further support to the literature around digital storytelling as a viable adjunctive to a traditional therapeutic process for coping with cancer-related stress in young people.

Background

Adolescent and young adult (AYA) oncology patients experience unique challenges that are not typically seen in other age groups (Stava et al., 2006). During this distinct period of development, AYAs are dealing with physical, cognitive, social, and emotional changes (Caskey & Anfara, 2007; Ogden & Hagen, 2018). A cancer diagnosis during this critical stage of growth can disrupt normal maturation (Park et al., 2018; Pereira

DOI: 10.4324/9781315622507-9

et al., 2020; Smith et al., 2013a, 2013b). Specifically, AYA cancer patients experience a disruption of schooling, socialization, and identity development (Patterson et al., 2012; Poort et al., 2018). Consequently, AYA oncology patients have been found to have poor mental health outcomes and low health-related quality of life (HRQOL), which can then impact overall health outcomes and HRQOL (Barnett et al., 2016; Smith et al., 2013a, 2013b; Varni et al., 1999). In this chapter, we aim to continue to identify how digital storytelling can provide a therapeutic release and aid in the processing of emotional distress for AYA cancer patients and survivors.

Literature has shown that the creation of expressive narratives is an effective therapeutic tool with many psychological and physiological benefits (Pennebaker & Chung, 2011; Taylor et al., 2016; Travagin et al., 2015). The process of engaging in expressive writing paradigms can decrease symptoms of distress due to medical illness and, in turn, improve overall health outcomes by addressing emotional inhibition that can put stress on the body (Baikie & Wilhelm, 2005; Pennebaker & Chung, 2011; Zakowski et al., 2004). Expressive narratives have also been found to promote healthy behaviors resulting in improved HRQOL (Hinyard & Kreuter, 2007; Pennebaker & Chung, 2011). Advances in modern technology and increased use of the web (e.g., YouTube and blogging) have led to the use of online narratives to express one's experiences with medical hardships (Chou et al., 2011; McBride, 2011). Despite recent advances in research around the therapeutic benefits of media-based narratives, such as those using video, for the AYA oncology population (Laing et al., 2017; Pereira et al., 2017), narrative filming is still a new concept. Therefore, the main objective of this chapter is to explore how the benefits of creating video narratives in the AYA oncology population may be experienced through utilizing language-based processes and how this may be translated to an intervention that will lead to emotional and physical benefits.

Literature Review

AYA Cancer Challenges

A growing body of literature surrounds the unique challenges that AYA cancer patients experience (Park et al., 2018; Poort et al., 2018; Zebrack et al., 2014). Beginning with diagnosis, AYA oncology patients experience disparities in medical treatment. Depending on age, the diagnosis, location of initial presentation for services, and hospital resources, AYAs are placed in either a pediatric or an adult cancer treatment center. Both environments are typically inadequate considering AYAs' developmental needs, either aiming too low or too high in age range (Pereira et al., 2020; Zebrack et al., 2014). Literature has also consistently shown that many AYA cancer patients feel their concerns regarding their physical changes and overall health are dismissed by healthcare providers (Patterson et al., 2017; Pereira et al., 2020). Sensitive topics such as sexual health changes and future implications for fertility are often overlooked (Murphy et al., 2013; Quinn et al., 2009). These unmet needs in medical treatment have resulted in poor mental health outcomes in AYA oncology patients (Park et al., 2018; Zebrack et al., 2014).

Poor mental health outcomes are also influenced by missing out on traditional social events and informal activities that healthy peers are engaging in (Jones et al., 2011; Pereira et al., 2020). Social interaction with peers during adolescence and young adulthood are critical to healthy development, especially around identity (a chief task of this developmental period) (Cai & Chaplin, 2019; Patterson et al., 2012). The inability to socialize or participate in social events with peers robs AYA patients of a key outlet for distraction and sources of social support (Cheung & Zebrack, 2017; Pereira et al., 2020). As a result, AYA oncology patients experience higher levels of traumatic stress and depressive symptoms than their healthy peers (Kazak et al., 2010; Sansom-Daly et al., 2018; Zakowski et al., 2004).

Modern Technology and Filmmaking

The creation of expressive narratives, including written and digital storytelling, is effective at helping AYA patients express and process trauma (Craft et al., 2012; Laing et al., 2017). Additionally, the use of film via vlogging to share one's experiences with mental health challenges as a way of educating others and gaining support has become increasingly popular among healthy AYAs and those suffering from mental illness (Peek et al., 2015; Pereira et al., 2016). The use of the internet and social media (YouTube, blogs, websites, video testimonials, vlogs) have been found to have a positive impact on individuals who have experienced trauma (Hoyt & Pasupathi, 2008; Mouthaan et al., 2011). A recent study conducted by Dobreski and Semaan (2017) revealed that video blogging is an effective coping mechanism for trauma associated with abuse or sexual assault. Likewise, therapeutic filmmaking has been found to promote hope and resilience in AYAs grieving the loss of a loved one (McGurl et al., 2015).

While there is a history of effective treatment using traditional psychotherapy for trauma (Goldbeck et al., 2016; Harmon, 1991; Martsolf & Draucker, 2005; Schneider et al., 2013), today's AYA oncology patients are more interested in nontraditional treatment methods, and these typically have better outcomes (Cheung & Zebrack, 2017). Due to illness-related barriers, many oncology patients experience social isolation and insufficient mental health services (Barnett et al., 2016; Park et al., 2018; Pereira et al., 2020). The use of film and social media is easily accessible and can be used as a tool to encourage positive mental health outcomes

(Johnson & Alderson, 2008; Kreuter et al., 2010; Laing et al., 2017). Eliciting video narratives allows AYAs to collect their thoughts and organize a story of their distressing experiences (Kreuter et al., 2010; Laing et al., 2017). A study conducted by Kreuter et al. (2010) revealed that the usage of video narratives led to increased communication between patients and their families. Additionally, sharing and watching other video narratives online has resulted in oncology patients and survivors feeling more connected with others and educated about their medical condition (Kreuter et al., 2010; Lang et al., 2020).

Why Do Digital and Video Narratives Work?

Considering limited resources and barriers during hospitalization, video narratives make an ideal and effective alternative method for engaging AYA patients who may be resistant to traditional psychotherapy (Johnson & Alderson, 2008; Pereira et al., 2020). Various types of digital interventions utilizing therapeutic methods are particularly helpful for individuals who experience difficulties associated with face-to-face services (Cohen & Mannarino, 2004; Johnson & Alderson, 2008; McCann et al., 2019). Additionally, a pilot study conducted by Johnson and Alderson (2008) that used a combination of traditional psychotherapy and therapeutic filmmaking was found to have better outcomes than traditional therapy alone. Participants reported filmmaking as being a better form of self-reflection and promoted autonomy regarding topics they wanted to discuss (Johnson & Alderson, 2008). These benefits reflect similar successes in traditional creative therapy that aim to encourage expression and facilitate the therapeutic process. With advances in modern technology, the internet has become widely used to promote psychological well-being (Forsman & Nordmyr, 2017). For the AYA oncology population, the internet can provide a place where AYAs can interact with their peers during times of forced social isolation due to medical restrictions (Chou & Moskowitz, 2016). A recent study found that the use of online chat groups following a viewing of video narratives facilitated emotion-focused group discussions in AYA oncology patients (Lang et al., 2020). Therapeutic benefits were seen through the process of connecting with group members and the ability to relate to and share their experiences (Lang et al., 2020). Additionally, it can be easier for many oncology patients and survivors to self-disclose online than in person, thus empowering patients who may not previously have had a voice around their care and experiences while also encouraging participation in traditional psychotherapy (Househ et al., 2014; Johnson & Alderson, 2008; McBride, 2011; Roberts, 2004).

Concerning the process of reciting one's narrative on film, expressive writing literature may provide the answer. Expressive writing has been used as a tool for promoting psychological well-being for nearly three decades (Craft et al., 2012; De Luca Picione et al., 2016; Smyth et al.,

2001; Stanton & Danoff-Burg, 2002). The process of written emotional disclosure has been found to aid in increasing emotional regulation, promoting optimistic thinking, and encouraging the use of coping skills (Campbell & Pennebaker, 2003; Giannotta et al., 2009; King, 2002; Lepore et al., 2002). A number of studies have shown expressive writing to be particularly beneficial for trauma recovery (Baddeley & Singer, 2008; Boals et al., 2011; Craft et al., 2012; Smyth et al., 2001). Given that AYA cancer patients and survivors often experience trauma associated with diagnosis and treatment (Zakowski et al., 2004), it is believed that expressive writing is particularly valuable for this population (Barnett et al., 2016; Park et al., 2018; Smith et al., 2013a, 2013b).

According to Morris and Shakespeare-Finch (2011), written narrative interventions in the oncology population were found to promote high levels of post-traumatic growth. The benefits of written narratives are thought to be a result of internal reflection that takes place following the writing process and is directly reflected in the language used in a writer's narrative (Craft et al., 2012; Habermas & de Silveira, 2008; McLean, 2005; Smyth et al., 2001). The key component of reflecting and processing one's experience is the organization and recoding of disorganized and avoidant thoughts that are typically associated with trauma, effectively acting as a form of exposure therapy (O'Kearney & Perrott, 2006; Smyth et al., 2001). This process of organizing and telling one's story brings unknown issues into the conscious mind, resulting in personal growth and meaning-making of the writer's experiences (Baikie & Wilhelm, 2005; Klein & Boals, 2001; Neimeyer, 2014). As such, narratives become more organized and reflect the resilience of the writer over time. The use of processing language in written narratives has been found to increase post-traumatic growth and promote overall improvements in quality of life (Alvarez-Conrad et al., 2001; Moore & Brody, 2009; Ullrich & Lutgendorf, 2002). It should then follow that video narratives offer an updated version of expressive writing for the modern age.

Current Study

Even though research on the usage of video narratives in the AYA oncology population is growing in popularity, it is still a limited research topic. To help continue to bridge this gap in the literature, in the present study we explored the psychological and physical benefits of creating video narratives in AYA cancer patients and survivors in the context of process-based language. Taking into account the literature mentioned earlier, we hypothesized the following:

H1: Resilient Qualities of the narrative, as identified by process-based language, will be higher in the second half of participants' video testimonials compared to the first half.

H2: Higher levels of Resilient Qualities of the narrative within the second half of video testimonials will predict higher scores on the Post Video Impressions Questionnaire (PVIQ) self-impact scale.

Methods

Recruitment and Participant Criteria

We collected data through the following institutions with IRB or Research Committee approval: Maria Farreri Children's Hospital, Children's Hospital of Orange County, Children's Hospital of Philadelphia, and Lucille Packard Children's Hospital of Stanford. Participants were recruited through flyer distribution, by phone recruitment, and through an in-person consultation with healthcare professionals. Participation criteria required individuals to be current cancer patients receiving treatment or childhood cancer survivors in remission for at least one year. All cancer diagnoses were included. Participants must have been diagnosed with cancer between the ages of 11 and 18 to participate.

Given the highly verbal nature of the study, participants whose cognitive and/or verbal capacities were limited due to illness or treatment were excluded from the study based on a cutoff result of one of the measures used. Other exclusionary criteria included participants treated for other chronic medical conditions prior to their cancer diagnosis. Questionnaires were administered in English, requiring participants to be proficient enough in the English language to read and understand the questions. Parental ability to read in English was not an exclusion factor, as parental consent was administered, as needed, via a translator.

Testing Procedure

Pre-video recording. Prior to the consent process, the Cognitive Log (Cog-Log) was given to determine cognitive-based eligibility for the study, assessing the participant's basic cognitive functioning and orientation. No individuals scored below the cutoff point, and all were able to proceed. Consent and assent were given accordingly based on the age group of the participant. Once consent/assent was obtained, parents were asked to leave the room, and participants completed a series of demographic questionnaires that also addressed cancer diagnosis, history of treatment, and experience with video narratives. Parents were later allowed to assist with any demographic questions which a participant was unable to answer due to uncertainty. In addition to demographics, participants completed the Health-Related Quality of Life (PedsQL), Ten-Item Personality Inventory (TIPI), and the Delis-Kaplan Executive Functioning System Verbal Fluency Test (D-KEFS).

Video recording. Following the questionnaires, participants were asked to recite their narratives and were read one of two prompts:

- *Prompt for participants with cancer*:

  "We'd like you to see what it would be like for you to make a YouTube video for others who want to know more about teens' experiences with cancer. Speak to the camera as if you were using your computer at home to make a video, and in detail, tell about your experiences since being diagnosed. Start at the beginning, include a middle, and end with where you are now. When you are done and would like to turn off the camera, let me know."

- *Prompt for survivors of cancer*:

  "We'd like to see what it would be like for you to make a YouTube video for others who want to know more about young people's experiences with cancer. Speak to the camera as if you were using your computer at home to make a video and, in detail, tell about your experiences as a cancer survivor. Start at the beginning (typically when you were diagnosed), include a middle, and end with where you are now. When you are done and would like to turn off the camera, let me know."

Participants were given time to prepare their narrative and ask the researcher questions. Once the participants were ready, the researcher presented the following options of visual self-disclosure for their video: being in full view of the camera, having a close-up of only their face and upper body on camera, having another body part of choice on camera (e.g., only showing feet), or having another object in the room on camera with only the participant's voice being recorded. The researcher then focused the camera per the participant's instruction and exited the room. The participant was advised to inform the researcher when the narrative was completed. If a participant was unable to turn on the camcorder due to physical restrictions, the researcher assisted before exiting the room. Participants were given privacy from researchers, parents, and others and recorded their narratives in an empty room, modeling a realistic recording environment free of observer-bias. Participants did not receive a time restraint on their recording. No editing took place, and no additional features were added to the videos once filming was complete. Following the completion of video recording, a researcher entered the room, turned off the recording if necessary, and administered the Post Video Impressions Questionnaire.

Measures

Cognitive Log (Cog-Log): The Cog-Log is a five- to ten-minute assessment measuring basic cognitive functioning and orientation, shown to have excellent validity and reliability (Alderson & Novack, 2003). The assessment was administered before the consent process. Scoring below the cut-off would indicate difficulty with verbal skills and/or the ability to understand the consent process and procedure of the study, thus excluding one from the study. In our study, no participants scored below the cutoff.

Post Video Impressions Questionnaire: The Post Video Impressions Questionnaire (PVIQ) was administered following completion of the narratives and served as a self-impact scale, measuring the following dimensions: the impact on the participant of making the video testimonial, the participant's perceived view of the impact the video might have on viewers, the desire to share the video online, the impact of reciting one's narrative on social relationships, the impact of reciting one's narrative on health-related behaviors, and the potential motivation for producing a video narrative to create a legacy (Pereira, 2017). See Table 6.1 for a full list of items. Scores on the PVIQ were used to examine the impact on participants of reciting their narrative and to construe the meaning behind their story.

Video Analyses

Following each testing session, the audio of each video recording was transcribed into a text file, reviewed by at least two more researchers for

Table 6.1 Dimensions of the Post Video Impressions Questionnaire

Dimensions	Items
Public video accessibility	I would post this video online for others to watch.
	I would place strong security settings on this video to control who watches it.
Perceived impact of watching the video on others; legacy; perceived impact on social relationships	Others watching this video would find it helpful.
Perceived impact of watching the video on others; perceived impact on social relationships	Others watching this video would find it upsetting.
	Others watching this video would feel something positive.
Perceived impact of watching the video on others; legacy	Others that watch this video may be professional staff who may be influenced to improve services to young people with cancer.
Perceived impact of watching the video on others; perceived impact on social relationships	If people I know watched this video, they would feel closer to me.
	If people watched this video, they would understand me better.
	If people watched this video, they would treat me differently.
Perceived impact of watching the video on others; legacy; perceived impact on social relationships	I said certain things in my video to help others.

(Continued)

Table 6.1 (Continued)

Dimensions	Items
Impact of creating the video on the participant	I said certain things in my video to help myself.
	After making this video, I felt sad.
	After making this video, I felt hopeful.
	After making this video, I felt happy.
	After making this video, I felt angry.
	After making this video, I felt relieved.
	After making this video, I felt stronger.
	After making this video, I learned something about myself.
	Making this video changed the way I think about my experiences with cancer.
	Making this video changed the way I think about my relationships with my healthcare team.
	After making this video, I will make another video about my experiences with cancer.
Impact of creating the video on the participant; perceived impact on social relationships	Making this video changed the way I think about my relationships with those close to me.
	Making this video made me feel closer to those I care about.
	After making this video, I plan on taking better care of others.
Impact of creating the video on the participant; change health-related behaviors	After making this video, I plan on taking better care of myself.
	After making this video, I will continue to find ways to express my feelings about my experiences with cancer.
Impact of creating the video on the participant; legacy	After making this video, I feel that I have made an important contribution to improving health programs for young people with cancer.
	After making this video, I feel that I have done something that will directly benefit other young people with cancer.

Note: Adapted from "Can making video testimonials benefit adolescents with cancer," by L. Pereira, Doc Diss 2017.

accuracy, and coded to determine the redemptive and resilient qualities of each participant using the Redemption Scale and coding categories from the (Linguistic Inquiry and Word Count program). To ensure reliability, members of the research team underwent a training exercise which consisted of coding eight random transcripts, reaching 88% reliability before continuing. All videos were destroyed following the final data analysis of the project except two to five videos selected with consent for future research and training purposes.

Redemption Level: The Redemption Scale, developed by Habermas and Diel, ranges from –2 to 2, with –2 being a story beginning positively but ending negatively and 2 being a story beginning negatively and ending positively (Habermas & Diel, 2013). These scores relate to a person's understanding of the impact of the event in question on their life's trajectory (i.e., this event impacted my life positively vs. negatively). A more positive view of the event has been linked to better emotional outcomes, higher health-related quality of life, and greater personal growth (McAdams et al., 2006). In this study, a higher redemption level suggests that the participant interpreted his or her illness throughout the narrative, making sense of the illness through a process of reappraisal.

LIWC—Linguistic Measure of Resilient Qualities of the Narrative: The Linguistic Inquiry and Word Count (LIWC) is a program developed by James Pennebaker et al. (2015) used to analyze the language in text files by processing each word individually and sorting them into separate functions or categories (Tausczik & Pennebaker, 2010). For the purpose of this study, each video narrative was transcribed and, using the LIWC, measured for resilient qualities within the narrative. Constructs related to resilience which were measured include narrator connectedness, narrative complexity, temporal distinction, and causal coherence. Each construct focuses on the function of words in relation to the overall narrative. A higher score on each construct suggests more resilient qualities.

- *Narrator connectedness* refers to how connected the narrator feels to their experience with illness and the role it plays in their story, measured by the use of singular first-person pronouns and insight words using LIWC. The ability to use first-person pronouns (e.g., *I*, *we*) versus second-person pronouns (e.g., *you*) shows a level of self-disclosure and personalization within the narrative, rather than distancing themselves from the narrative through second-person pronouns (Tausczik & Pennebaker, 2010).

- *Narrative complexity* is related to both thematic content and language complexity within the narrative, measured by prepositions (e.g., *with, for, on*), cognitive mechanism words (e.g., *should cause*), and words with 6+ letters (Tausczik & Pennebaker, 2010). The type of words chosen by the narrator and the process language used show insight into how the narrator makes sense of his or her story throughout the video narrative (Burke & Dollinger, 2005).

- *Temporal distinction* refers to the order of the narrative in which the narrator is able to tell his or her story from beginning, middle, to end in a linear sequence while providing depth in the meaning of the content. This was measured through differentiation words, which provide a distinction between categories, and through conjunctions (e.g., *and, although, also, but*) which serve to join separate segments of the story to give order to the narrative (Tausczik & Pennebaker, 2010).

- The use of *causal words* (e.g., *because, hence*) and insight words (e.g., *think, know, consider*) measure causal coherence, which suggests a deeper quality of the meaning behind the narrative and an active process of reappraisal in which the narrator uses process language to reexamine their experience as they are narrating (Burke & Dollinger, 2005; Tausczik & Pennebaker, 2010). This cognitive reappraisal unfolds an understanding of the meaning of separate events described by the narrator and puts it in perspective within the overall narrative.

Results

Demographics

The final study sample consisted of 24 cancer patients and 8 cancer survivors between 12 and 41 years of age, with the average age being 17 years. There were 17 females (53%) and 15 males (47%), for a total of 32 participants. Age of diagnosis ranged from 11 to 18 years of age, with a mean of 14 years of age. Types of cancer included blood cancer (59.4%), central nervous system (CNS) cancer (9.4%), and solid tumors (31.3%). Days since diagnosis ranged from 30 to 9,490 days, with a mean of 1,254 days. Self-reported race and ethnicity were as follows: Asian (12.5%), Hispanic (40.6%), Mixed Race (15.6%), and White (31.3%). All 32 participants were included in analyses for the first hypothesis; however, only 31 participants were included in the analyses for the second hypothesis, as a 17-year-old male with a blood cancer was excluded because he did not complete the PVIQ.

Main Analyses

We first hypothesized that resilient qualities of the narrative would be higher in the second half of participants' video testimonials compared to the first half. After dividing the narrative transcripts in half, paired samples t-tests with a one-tailed significance were conducted comparing Causal Coherence, Narrator Connectedness, Narrative Complexity, and Temporal Distinction in the first versus second half of the transcript. Results indicated there was a significant difference in resilient qualities, as measured by Narrator Connectedness, in the first half of the narrative (M = 13.62, SD = 2.38) versus the second half of the narrative (M = 12.5, SD = 2.99); $t(31)$ = 2.08, p = .02. However, this indicated a decrease from the first to the second half. We ran post hoc analyses to compare additional LIWC variables related to cognitive processing and potential time of reference so as to better understand these results. Results indicated cognitive processing was higher in the second half of the narrative (M = 14.34, SD = 3.48) than the first half

(M = 12.33, SD = 2.94); $t(31) = -2.93$, $p = .00$. Further results showed process-based language was higher in the second half of the narrative with regard to causation ($t(31) = -2.50$, $p = .01$), tentativeness ($t(31) = -1.83$, $p = .04$), certainty ($t(31) = -2.87$, $p = .00$), and differentiation ($t(31) = .392$, $p = .00$). Participants also focused more on the present in the second half of the narrative (M = 12.95, SD = 3.67) than the first half (M = 7.99, SD = 2.64); $t(31)-7.22$, $p = .00$. In the first half of the narrative, participants were more focused on the past ($(t)7.57$, $p = .00$) and used more insight words ($t(31) = .93$, $p = .00$). See Table 6.2 for full results.

We also hypothesized that higher levels of resilient qualities of the narrative within the second half of the video testimonials would predict higher scores on the PVIQ self-impact scale (H2). A stepwise regression analysis was conducted to predict scores on the PVIQ self-impact scale based on resilient qualities through Causal Coherence, Narrator Connectedness, and Narrative Complexity, controlling for time since diagnosis. Results indicated Narrator Connectedness was a significant predictor of positive impact from reciting one's narrative on film ($t = 2.91$, $p = .00$). See Table 6.3 for full results.

Table 6.2 Paired Samples t-Test Results Between First Half of Narrative and Second Half of Narrative

Variable	First Half		Second Half			
	M	*SD*	*M*	*SD*	*t(31)*	*One tailed p-value*
Narrator Connectedness	13.62	2.38	12.5	2.99	2.08	0.02
Narrator Complexity	36.82	2.97	37.49	4.55	−0.68	0.25
Temporal Distinction	13.76	1.96	14.54	2.65	−1.99	0.03
Causal Coherence	4.3	1.51	4.52	1.83	−0.57	0.29
Cognitive Processing	12.33	2.94	14.34	3.47	−2.93	0.00
Insight	2.93	1.12	2.65	1.56	0.93	0.18
Causation	1.37	0.84	1.88	0.81	−2.5	0.01
Discrepancies	1.28	0.81	1.48	0.84	−1.18	0.12
Tentative	2.43	1.33	2.9	1.42	−1.83	0.04
Certainty	1.41	0.88	1.89	1.14	−2.87	0.00
Differentiation	3.65	1.18	4.67	1.65	−3.92	0.00
Past Focus	9.56	2.23	5.97	2.46	7.57	0.00
Present Focus	7.99	2.64	12.95	3.67	−7.22	0.00
Future Focus	1.49	1.11	1.8	1.16	−2.95	0.00

Table 6.3 Predictors of Scores on the PVIQ Self-Impact Scale

Variable	n	B	SE	β	t	One tailed p-value
Redemption Level	32	2.22	1.92	0.23	1.16	0.13
Causal Coherence	32	0.85	1.35	0.13	0.63	0.27
Narrator Connectedness	32	2.21	0.76	0.57	2.91	0.00
Narrative Complexity	32	-0.27	0.74	-0.1	-0.36	0.36
Temporal Distinction	32	0.07	0.99	0.02	0.07	0.47
Cognitive Processing	32	-0.46	0.72	-0.13	-0.64	0.26
Insight	32	3.98	1.81	0.5	2.2	0.02
Causation	32	-0.41	3.21	-0.03	-0.13	0.45
Discrepancies	32	4.98	3.43	0.31	1.45	0.08
Tentative	32	-3.06	2.95	-0.38	-1.04	0.16
Certainty	32	5.31	4.05	0.36	1.31	0.10
Differentiation	32	-5.51	5.33	-0.69	-1.03	0.16

Note: $N = 32$.

Discussion

Results of this study partially support our hypothesis that the second portion of an AYA patient or survivor's digital cancer narrative will contain more process-based language and thus lead to a greater benefit in reciting their narrative. It is not uncommon for chronically ill patients, especially those diagnosed with cancer, to be asked to share their stories for others. However, these stories are often rehearsed and focus on the diagnosis and treatment process with a "nugget" at the end to reflect the strength or growth of the narrator. In the case of our study participants, data suggested that the first half of the narrative, which typically focuses on diagnosis and treatment, did present a straightforward timeline of factual information. However, the second half contained more process-based language and focused on the self. This process confirms suspicions that after reciting a well-rehearsed history of their cancer story, AYAs switch to more reflection on their experiences and begin to explore their trauma.

During the debriefing process of this study, a few participants noted that participating in this study was the first time they were able to tell their story for themselves, without needing to find a "good sound bite." Several also noted that they had never shared their story in its completion out loud before. It would then make sense for narratives during the second half to lack a significantly higher level of resilient qualities, as these qualities suggest a narrative that is well formed and thus trauma that has already been processed. Additionally, the time focus of the narrative changed from past to present, which we assume (in addition to the current state of their lives) includes discussion around a patient's current feelings and beliefs about their experience. Our films suggest that when given the space to talk freely and openly, AYA patients eventually begin to talk in a stream of consciousness and actively process on camera. This reflects earlier findings by Laing et al. (2017) that may differ from the expressive writing process, as writing slows down the ability to reflect on topics in the moment.

This data also included both patients and survivors. Time since treatment was controlled for in the second hypothesis. However, it was found to be significant in predicting the benefit of reciting one's narrative on film. We did not have enough data to separate each group. This finding suggests that while certain circumstances for patients predict a benefit in reciting their narrative, survivors may universally benefit from sharing their narrative. It is possible that this is due to their stage of life and history with their cancer. In an earlier evaluation of this data, patients with a more severe course of treatment struggled with sharing their story on film (Pereira, 2017). It was suggested that this was due to confronting the reality of their experiences for the first time after being in "survival mode" for an extended period. Survivors, on the other hand, may relish the ability to finally confront their cancer history after avoiding it for so long.

Limitations

This study population included both patients and survivors. While this allows for generalizability of the data, it also introduces one's life history with cancer as a confounding variable. Even though time since diagnosis was controlled for, survivors have had more experience with cancer. Along with that experience may come grappling with late effects, seeing other friends pass away from the disease, potentially experiencing a relapse themselves, and a number of other influences of cancer on one's life. A larger survivor sample is therefore needed to tease out group differences.

Future Directions

We used this data to look at the overall benefit of reciting one's narrative on film; however, additional analyses from the PVIQ are available. We can also examine perceived benefits that others may experience from watching digital narratives, personal health benefits, and possible social benefits. While earlier analyses have suggested universal benefits to reciting one's cancer narrative on film, differences emerge when looking at motivation for content (Pereira, 2017). Specifically, while AYA cancer patients do recognize that others can benefit from watching the film, there is a greater focus on themselves compared to healthy peers who may share difficult experiences so that others can understand them. Understanding these benefits specific to process-based language and potential post-traumatic growth will shed light on more of the potential benefits patients may experience.

As previously stated, more research is needed on AYA cancer survivors' experiences with digital storytelling. In addition to a greater focus on how survivors differ from patients in *why* digital narratives are beneficial, *how* their language and thus processing is different from patients will also shed light on the psychological state of AYA cancer survivors. This may, in turn, help clinicians determine better interventions for this group of survivors. Research has found that AYA survivors of pediatric and AYA cancer lag significantly behind their healthy peers around a number of milestones, including the ability to live fulfilling, independent lives (Duijts et al., 2013). Interventions that support post-traumatic growth and positive HRQOL outcomes are needed.

While this study paradigm is in some ways modeled after expressive writing, expressive writing relies on the patient to process their written narrative after its completion and in between writing sessions. In contrast, this study has shown that AYA oncology patients and survivors are processing their trauma story while reciting it. Further research is needed to truly tease out the different processes involved in creating digital narratives and to compare them directly, as an intervention, to expressive writing.

Lastly, research to understand how these narratives are used online is needed as well. While items are asked on the PVIQ to identify how participants might share their film online, this subset of data did not explore its connection to language and benefits experienced for participants. Previous data has shown mixed results with specific factors influencing this (e.g., personality type and amount of self-disclosure) (Pereira, 2017; Pereira & Braniecki, 2017; Pereira et al., 2018). Research has suggested that online communities that use digital narratives are helpful to survivors (Chou et al., 2011), but more vigorous research is needed to target how this kind of intervention can be used safely to maximize patient benefits.

Conclusion

A series of studies from this lab, as well as others, have now established that Adolescent and Young Adult cancer patients and survivors, as well as other young people, can benefit from sharing their cancer stories on film. Whether this intervention can be translated to a traditional therapeutic process and integrated as well as its other creative therapy partners is still under ongoing investigation. However, anecdotal evidence from patients during the debriefing process would suggest otherwise. In particular, while reflecting on her participation in the study, one participant stated she had an upcoming psychotherapy appointment, and she had a lot more she needed to share with her therapist. It is the hope of the study team that more comments like this will be made, and digital narratives will increasingly help young people open up to others and continue to share their stories to support their personal growth and well-being.

References

Alderson, A. L., & Novack, T. A. (2003). Reliable serial measurement of cognitive processes in rehabilitation: The cognitive log. *Archives of Physical Medicine and Rehabilitation, 84*(5), 668–672. doi: 10.1016/s0003-9993(02)04842-6

Alvarez-Conrad, J., Zoellner, L. A., & Foa, E. B. (2001). Linguistic predictors of trauma pathology and physical health. *Applied Cognitive Psychology: The Official Journal of the Society for Applied Research in Memory and Cognition, 15*(7), S159–S170. doi: 10.1002/acp.839

Baddeley, J. L., & Singer, J. A. (2008). Telling losses: Personality correlates and functions of bereavement narratives. *Journal of Research in Personality, 42*(2), 421–438. doi: 10.1016/j.jrp.2007.07.006

Baikie, K. A., & Wilhelm, K. (2005). Emotional and physical health benefits of expressive writing. *Advances in Psychiatric Treatment, 11*(5), 338–346. doi: 10.1192/apt.11.5.338

Barnett, M., McDonnell, G., DeRosa, A., Schuler, T., Philip, E., Peterson, L., Touza, K., Jhanwar, S., Atkinson, T. M., & Ford, J. S. (2016). Psychosocial outcomes and interventions among cancer survivors diagnosed during adolescence and young adulthood (AYA): A systematic review. *Journal of Cancer Survivorship, 10*(5), 814–831. doi: 10.1007/s11764-016-0527-6

Boals, A., Banks, J. B., Hathaway, L. M., & Schuettler, D. (2011). Coping with stressful events: Use of cognitive words in stressful narratives and the meaning-making process. *Journal of Social and Clinical Psychology, 30*(4), 378–403. doi: 10.1521/jscp.2011.30.4.378

Burke, P. A., & Dollinger, S. J. (2005). "A picture's worth a thousand words": Language use in the autophotographic essay. *Personality & Social Psychology Bulletin, 31*(4), 536–548. doi: 10.1177/0146167204271714

Cai, R. A., & Chaplin, H. (2019). Impact of rheumatic musculoskeletal disease on psychological development in adolescents and young adults. In J. E. McDonagh & R. S. Tattersall (Eds.), *Adolescent and young adult rheumatology in clinical practice* (pp. 19–34). Springer.

Campbell, R. S., & Pennebaker, J. W. (2003). The secret life of pronouns: Flexibility in writing style and physical health. *Psychological Science, 14*(1), 60–65. doi: 10.1111/1467-9280.01419

Caskey, M. M., & Anfara Jr., V. A. (2007). Research summary: Young adolescents' developmental characteristics. *National Middle School Association.* http://archives.pdx.edu/ds/psu/9578

Cheung, C. K., & Zebrack, B. (2017). What do adolescents and young adults want from cancer resources? Insights from a Delphi panel of AYA patients. *Supportive Care in Cancer, 25*(1), 119–126. doi: 10.1007/s00520-016-3396-7

Chou, W.-Y. S., Hunt, Y., Folkers, A., & Augustson, E. (2011). Cancer survivorship in the age of YouTube and social media: A narrative analysis. *Journal of Medical Internet Research*, *13*(1), e7. doi: 10.2196/jmir.1569

Chou, W.-Y. S., & Moskowitz, M. (2016). Social media use in adolescent and young adult (AYA) cancer survivors. *Current Opinion in Psychology*, *9*, 88–91. https://www.dhi.ac.uk/san/waysofbeing/data/health-jones-chou-2016.pdf

Cohen, J. A., & Mannarino, A. P. (2004). Treatment of childhood traumatic grief. *Journal of Clinical Child and Adolescent Psychology*, *33*(4), 819–831. doi: 10.1207/s15374424jccp3304_17

Craft, M. A., Davis, G. C., & Paulson, R. M. (2012). Expressive writing in early breast cancer survivors. *Journal of Advanced Nursing*, *69*(2), 305–315. doi: 10.1111/j.1365-2648.2012.06008.x

De Luca Picione, R., Martino, M. L., & Freda, M. F. (2016). Understanding cancer patients' narratives: Meaning-making process, temporality, and modal articulation. *Journal of Constructivist Psychology*, *30*(4), 339–359. doi: 10.1080/10720537.2016.1227738

Dobreski, B., & Semaan, B. (2017). Blogging as recovery: The use of blogs by survivors of military sexual trauma. *Proceedings of the Association for Information Science and Technology*, *54*(1), 652–654. doi: 10.1002/pra2.2017.14505401103

Duijts, S. F. A., van Egmond, M. P., Spelten, E., van Muijen, P., Anema, J. R., & van der Beek, A. J. (2013), Physical and psychosocial problems in cancer survivors beyond return to work: A systematic review. *Psycho-Oncology*, *23*, 481–492. doi: 10.1002/pon.3467

Forsman, A. K., & Nordmyr, J. (2017). Psychosocial links between Internet use and mental health in later life: A systematic review of quantitative and qualitative evidence. *Journal of Applied Gerontology*, *36*(12), 1471–1518. doi: 10.1177/0733464815595509

Giannotta, F., Settanni, M., Kliewer, W., & Ciairano, S. (2009). Results of an Italian school-based expressive writing intervention trial focused on peer problems. *Journal of Adolescence*, *32*(6), 1377–1389. doi: 10.1016/j.adolescence.2009.07.001

Goldbeck, L., Muche, R., Sachser, C., Tutus, D., & Rosner, R. (2016). Effectiveness of trauma-focused cognitive behavioral therapy for children and adolescents: A randomized controlled trial in eight German mental health clinics. *Psychotherapy and Psychosomatics*, *85*(3), 159–170. doi: 10.1159/000442824

Habermas, T., & de Silveira, C. (2008). The development of global coherence in life narratives across adolescence: Temporal, causal, and thematic aspects. *Developmental Psychology*, *44*(3), 707–721. doi: 10.1037/0012-1649.44.3.707

Habermas, T., & Diel, V. (2013). The episodicity of verbal reports of personally significant autobiographical memories: Vividness correlates with narrative text quality more than with detailedness or memory specificity. *Frontiers in Behavioral Neuroscience*, *7*, 110. doi: 10.3389/fnbeh.2013.00110

Harmon, M. J. (1991). The use of group psychotherapy with cancer patients: A review of recent literature. *Journal for Specialists in Group Work*, *16*(1), 56–61. doi: 10.1080/01933929108415587

Hinyard, L. J., & Kreuter, M. W. (2007). Using narrative communication as a tool for health behavior change: A conceptual, theoretical, and empirical overview. *Health Education & Behavior*, *34*(5), 777–792. doi: 10.1177/1090198106291963

Househ, M., Borycki, E., & Kushniruk, A. (2014). Empowering patients through social media: The benefits and challenges. *Health Informatics Journal*, 20(1), 50–58. doi: 10.1177/1460458213476969

Hoyt, T., & Pasupathi, M. (2008). Blogging about trauma: Linguistic markers of apparent recovery. *E-Journal of Applied Psychology*, 4(2), 56–62. doi: 10.7790/ejap.v4i2.106

Johnson, J. L., & Alderson, K. G. (2008). Therapeutic filmmaking: An exploratory pilot study. *The Arts in Psychotherapy*, 35(1), 11–19. doi: 10.1016/j.aip.2007.08.004

Jones, B. L., Parker-Raley, J., & Barczyk, A. (2011). Adolescent cancer survivors: Identity paradox and the need to belong. *Qualitative Health Research*, 21(8), 1033–1040. doi: 10.1177/1049732311404029

Kazak, A. E., DeRosa, B. W., Schwartz, L. A., Hobbie, W., Carlson, C., Ittenbach, R. F., Mao, J. J., & Ginsberg, J. P. (2010). Psychological outcomes and health beliefs in adolescent and young adult survivors of childhood cancer and controls. *Journal of Clinical Oncology*, 28(12), 2002–2007. doi: 10.1200/JCO.2009.25.9564

King, L. A. (2002). *Gain without pain? Expressive writing and self-regulation.* In S. J. Lepore & J. M. Smyth (Eds.), *The writing cure: How expressive writing promotes health and emotional well-being* (pp. 119–134). American Psychological Association. doi: 10.1037/10451-006

Klein, K., & Boals, A. (2001). The relationship of life event stress and working memory capacity. *Applied Cognitive Psychology: The Official Journal of the Society for Applied Research in Memory and Cognition*, 15(5), 565–579. doi: 10.1002/acp.727

Kreuter, M. W., Holmes, K., Alcaraz, K., Kalesan, B., Rath, S., Richert, M., McQueen, A. Caito, N., Robinson, L., & Clark, E. M. (2010). Comparing narrative and informational videos to increase mammography in low-income African American women. *Patient Education and Counseling*, 81(Suppl), S6–S14. doi: 10.1016/j.pec.2010.09.008

Laing, C. M., Moules, N. J., Estefan, A., & Lang, M. (2017). Stories that heal: Understanding the effects of creating digital stories with pediatric and adolescent/young adult oncology patients. *Journal of Pediatric Oncology Nursing*, 34(4), 272–282. doi: 10.1177/1043454216688639

Lang, M. J., Dort, J. C., Stephen, J., Lamont, L., & Giese-Davis, J. (2020). Narrative-informed emotion-focused psychotherapy in synchronous, online chat groups for adolescents and young adults with cancer: A proof-of-concept study. *Journal of Adolescent and Young Adult Oncology*, 9(6), 676–682. doi: 10.1089/jayao.2020.0030

Lepore, S. J., Greenberg, M. A., Bruno, M., & Smyth, J. M. (2002). Expressive writing and health: Self-regulation of emotion-related experience, physiology, and behavior. In S. J. Lepore & J. M. Smyth (Eds.), *The writing cure: How expressive writing promotes health and emotional well-being* (pp. 99–117). American Psychological Association. doi: 10.1037/10451-005

Martsolf, D. S., & Draucker, C. B. (2005). Psychotherapy approaches for adult survivors of childhood sexual abuse: An integrative review of outcomes research. *Issues in Mental Health Nursing*, 26(8), 801–825. doi: 10.1080/01612840500184012

McAdams, D. P., Bauer, J. J., Sakaeda, A. R., Anyidoho, N. A., Machado, M. A., Magrino-Failla, K., White, K. W., & Pals, J. L. (2006). Continuity and change in the life story: A longitudinal study of autobiographical memories in emerging adulthood. *Journal of Personality, 74*(5), 1371–1400. doi: 10.1111/j.1467-6494.2006.00412.x

McBride, D. (2011). Cancer survivors find blogging improves quality of life. *ONS Connect, 26*(4), 20. https://rucreativebloggingfa13.files.wordpress.com/2013/09/cancersurvivorsblogging.pdf

McCann, L., McMillan, K. A., & Pugh, G. (2019). Digital interventions to support adolescents and young adults with cancer: Systematic review. *JMIR Cancer, 5*(2), e12071. doi: 10.2196/12071

McGurl, C., Seegobin, W., Hamilton, E., & McMinn, M. (2015). The benefits of a grief and loss program with a unique technological intervention. In J. L. Cohen, J. L. Johnson, & Orr, P. P. (Eds.), *Video and filmmaking as psychotherapy: Research and practice* (pp. 81–94). Routledge.

McLean, K. C. (2005). Late adolescent identity development: Narrative meaning making and memory telling. *Developmental Psychology, 41*(4), 683–691. doi: 10.1037/0012-1649.41.4.683

Moore, S. D., & Brody, L. R. (2009). Linguistic predictors of mindfulness in written self-disclosure narratives. *Journal of Language and Social Psychology, 28*(3), 281–296. doi: 10.1177/0261927X09335264

Morris, B. A., & Shakespeare-Finch, J. (2011). Cancer diagnostic group differences in posttraumatic growth: Accounting for age, gender, trauma severity, and distress. *Journal of Loss and Trauma, 16*(3), 229–242. doi: 10.1080/15325024.2010.519292

Mouthaan, J., Sijbrandij, M., Reitsma, J., Gersons, B. R., & Olff, M. (2011). Internet-based prevention of posttraumatic stress symptoms in injured trauma patients: Design of a randomized controlled trial. *European Journal of Psychotraumatology, 2*(1), Article 8294. doi: 10.3402/ejpt.v2i0.8294

Murphy, D., Orgel, E., Termuhlen, A., Shannon, S., Warren, K., & Quinn, G. P. (2013). Why healthcare providers should focus on the fertility of AYA cancer survivors: It's not too late! *Frontiers in Oncology, 3*, 248. doi: 10.3389/fonc.2013.00248

Neimeyer, R. (2014). Re-storying loss: Fostering growth in the posttraumatic narrative. In L. G. Calhoun & R. G. Tedeschi (Eds.), *Handbook of posttraumatic growth: Research and practice* (pp. 82–94). Routledge.

O'Kearney, R., & Perrott, K. (2006). Trauma narratives in posttraumatic stress disorder: A review. *Journal of Traumatic Stress, 19*(1), 81–93. doi: 10.1002/jts.20099

Ogden, T., & Hagen, K. A. (2018). *Adolescent mental health: Prevention and intervention* (2nd ed.). Routledge.

Park, J. L., Brandelli, Y., Russell, K. B., Reynolds, K., Li, Y., Ruether, D., & Giese-Davis, J. (2018). Unmet needs of adult survivors of childhood cancers: Associations with developmental stage at diagnosis, cognitive impairment, and time from diagnosis. *Journal of Adolescent and Young Adult Oncology, 7*(1), 61–71. doi: 10.1089/jayao.2017.0023

Patterson, P., McDonald, F. E. J., White, K. J., Walczak, A., & Butow, P. N. (2017). Levels of unmet needs and distress amongst adolescents and young adults (AYAs) impacted by familial cancer. *Psycho-Oncology, 26*(9), 1285–1292. doi: 10.1002/pon.4421

Patterson, P., Millar, B., Desille, N., & McDonald, F. (2012). The unmet needs of emerging adults with a cancer diagnosis: A qualitative study. *Cancer Nursing*, *35*(3), E32–E40. doi: 10.1089/jayao.2017.0023

Peek, H. S., Richards, M., Muir, O., Chan, S. R., Caton, M., & MacMillan, C. (2015). Blogging and social media for mental health education and advocacy: A review for psychiatrists. *Current Psychiatry Reports*, *17*(11), Article 88. doi: 10.1007/s11920-015-0629-2

Pennebaker, J. W., Booth, R. J., Boyd, R. L., & Francis, M. E. (2015). *Linguistic inquiry and word count: LIWC2015.* [Computer software]. Pennebaker Conglomerates.

Pennebaker, J. W., & Chung, C. K. (2011). Expressive writing: Connections to physical and mental health. In H. S. Friedman (Ed.), *The Oxford handbook of health psychology* (pp. 417–437). Oxford University Press. doi: 10.1093/oxfordhb/9780195342819.013.0018

Pereira, L. (2017). *Can making video narratives benefit adolescents with cancer?* [Doctoral dissertation, Palo Alto University]. ProQuest Dissertations Publishing. [10288231] https://www.proquest.com/docview/1978076755?pq-origsite=gscholar&fromopenview=true

Pereira, L., Schmidt, M., & Tannenbaum, A. (2018, April). *The relationship between disclosure and impact of reciting a video narrative in adolescents with cancer and healthy peers.* Poster presented at the *Society for Pediatric Psychology Annual Conference, Orlando, FL.*

Pereira, L. M., & Braniecki, S. (2017, December). *Factors influencing visual and verbal self- disclosure of video narratives in teenagers with cancer: A pilot study.* Poster Presented at the *2nd Annual Global Adolescent and Young Adult Cancer Congress, Atlanta, GA.*

Pereira, L. M., Muench, A., & Lawton, B. (2017). The impact of making a video cancer narrative in an adolescent male: A case study. *The Arts in Psychotherapy*, *55*, 195–201. doi: 10.1016/j.aip.2017.06.004

Pereira, L. M., Piela, G., & DiCola, K. (2020). Thematic content of video narratives in patients and survivors of adolescent cancer. *Psycho-Oncology*, *29*(4), 759–765. doi: 10.1002/pon.5340

Pereira, L. M., Quinn, N., & Morales, E. (2016, October). Breaking news: "I have an eating disorder." Video testimonials on YouTube. *Computers in Human Behavior*, *63*, 938–942. doi: 10.1016/j.chb.2016.06.027

Poort, H., Souza, P. M., Malinowski, P. K., MacDougall, K. M., Barysauskas, C. M., Lau Greenberg, T., Tulsky, J. A., & Fasciano, K. M. (2018). Taking a "snapshot": Evaluation of a conversation aid for identifying psychosocial needs in young adults with cancer. *Journal of Adolescent and Young Adult Oncology*, *7*(5), 565–571. doi: 10.1089/jayao.2018.0027

Quinn, G. P., Vadaparampil, S. T., Lee, J.-H., Jacobsen, P. B., Bepler, G., Lancaster, J., Keefe, D. L., & Albrecht, T. L. (2009). Physician referral for fertility preservation in oncology patients: A national study of practice behaviors. *Journal of Clinical Oncology*, *27*(35), 5952–5957. doi: 10.1200/JCO.2009.23.0250

Roberts, P. (2004). The living and the dead: Community in the virtual cemetery. *OMEGA: Journal of Death and Dying*, *49*(1), 57–76. doi: 10.2190/D41T-YFNN-109K-WR4C

Sansom-Daly, U. M., Wakefield, C. E., Robertson, E. G., McGill, B. C., Wilson, H. L., & Bryant, R. A. (2018). Adolescent and young adult cancer survivors' memory and future thinking processes place them at risk for poor mental health. *Psycho-Oncology*, *27*(12), 2709–2716. doi: 10.1002/pon.4856

Schneider, S. J., Grilli, S. F., & Schneider, J. R. (2013). Evidence-based treatments for traumatized children and adolescents. *Current Psychiatry Reports, 15*(1), 332. doi: 10.1007/s11920-012-0332-5

Smith, A. W., Bellizzi, K. M., Keegan, T. H., Zebrack, B., Chen, V. W., Neale, A. V., Hamilton, S., Shnorhavorian, M., & Lynch, C. F. (2013a). Health-related quality of life of adolescent and young adult patients with cancer in the United States: The Adolescent and Young Adult Health Outcomes and Patient Experience study. *Journal of Clinical Oncology: Official Journal of the American Society of Clinical Oncology, 31*(17), 2136–2145. doi: 10.1200/JCO.2012.47.3173

Smith, A. W., Parsons, H. M., Kent, E. E., Bellizzi, K. M., Zebrack, B. J., Keel, G., Lynch, C. F., Rubenstein, M. B., Keegan, T. H., & AYA HOPE Study Collaborative Group. (2013b). Unmet support service needs and health-related quality of life among adolescents and young adults with cancer: The AYA HOPE study. *Frontiers in Oncology, 3*, Article 00075. doi: 10.3389/fonc.2013.00075

Smyth, J., True, N., & Souto, J. (2001). Effects of writing about traumatic experiences: The necessity for narrative structuring. *Journal of Social and Clinical Psychology, 20*(2), 161–172. doi: 10.1521/jscp.20.2.161.22266

Stanton, A. L., & Danoff-Burg, S. (2002). Emotional expression, expressive writing, and cancer. In S. J. Lepore & J. M. Smyth (Eds.), *The writing cure: How expressive writing promotes health and emotional well-being* (pp. 31–51). American Psychological Association. doi: 10.1037/10451-002

Stava, C. J., Lopez, A., & Vassilopoulou-Sellin, R. (2006). Health profiles of younger and older breast cancer survivors. *Cancer, 107*(8), 1752–1759. doi: 10.1002/cncr.22200

Tausczik, Y. R., & Pennebaker, J. W. (2010). The psychological meaning of words: LIWC and computerized text analysis methods. *Journal of Language & Social Psychology, 29*(10), 24–54. doi: 10.1177/0261927X09351676

Taylor, E., Jouriles, E. N., Brown, R., Goforth, K., & Banyard, V. (2016). Narrative writing exercises for promoting health among adolescents: Promises and pitfalls. *Psychology of Violence, 6*(1), 57–63. doi: 10.1037/vio0000023

Travagin, G., Margola, D., & Revenson, T. A. (2015). How effective are expressive writing interventions for adolescents? A meta-analytic review. *Clinical Psychology Review, 36*(1), 42–55. doi: 10.1016/j.cpr.2015.01.003

Ullrich, P. M., & Lutgendorf, S. K. (2002). Journaling about stressful events: Effects of cognitive processing and emotional expression. *Annals of Behavioral Medicine, 24*(3), 244–250. doi: 10.1207/S15324796ABM2403_10

Varni, J., Seid, M., & Rode, C. (1999). The PedsQL: Measurement model for the Pediatric Quality of Life Inventory. *Medical Care, 37*(20), 126–139. doi: 10.1097/00005650-199902000-00003

Zakowski, S. G., Ramati, A., Morton, C., Johnson, P., & Flanigan, R. (2004). Written emotional disclosure buffers the effects of social constraints on distress among cancer patients. *Health Psychology, 23*(6), 555–563. doi: 10.1037/0278-6133.23.6.555

Zebrack, B., Kent, E. E., Keegan, T. H., Kato, I., Smith, A. W., & AYA HOPE Study Collaborative Group. (2014). "Cancer sucks," and other ponderings by adolescent and young adult cancer survivors. *Journal of Psychosocial Oncology, 32*(1), 1–15. doi: 10.1080/07347332.2013.855959

7 Creating Impact through Trauma-Informed Drama Therapy using Videos and Films

The Efficacy of Purposeful Performance

Brooke Campbell

Introduction

In this chapter, I identify various trauma-informed drama therapy-based films, videos, and drama therapy programs which utilize film and video effectively and with intention. I also illustrate how film and video can be utilized as an educational, research, advocacy, and therapeutic tool which leads to positive outcomes and results. Interviews with well-known trauma-informed drama therapists who have utilized film and video in their work with trauma survivors are shared and highlighted. Positive outcomes can be seen with the survivors of trauma, families, organizations, and communities. This chapter focuses on trauma-informed drama therapy-based films, videos, programs, and the drama therapy methods utilized to explore how trauma can be healed, be transformed, and create lasting change along with positive social impact for our communities and the world at large.

Trauma and the Body

At the time of this writing, we are living through the historical pandemic of 2020. Trauma affects us all. Some various forms of trauma include individual, institutional, and collective trauma. What we are experiencing at this moment in time due to the spread of the coronavirus, or COVID-19, is most assuredly a collective trauma. Trauma psychologist Alaa Hijaz writes about the pandemic caused by the coronavirus:

> We are going through a collective trauma, that is bringing up profound grief, loss, panic over livelihoods, panic over loss of lives of loved ones. People's nervous systems are barely coping with the sense of threat and vigilance for safety, or alternating with feeling numb and frozen and shutting down in response to it all.
>
> (Reneau, 2020)

DOI: 10.4324/9781315622507-10

Trauma is stored in the body and yet we live in a world where there is much emphasis on using our cognitive abilities to heal. We cannot reason or rationalize or make sense of trauma or a traumatic experience by merely thinking about it or trying to make sense of it. Trauma causes fragmentation of one's memories and events. Oftentimes, trauma survivors will note in sessions not recalling or remembering the sequential details of the traumatic event they experienced. A metaphor used within my work with survivors of trauma likens a traumatic experience to a puzzle with all the pieces strewn everywhere due to memory gaps. The healing of trauma includes trying to put the entire puzzle together to create a cohesively whole image with a linear timeline to process and make sense of what happened.

Dr. Sandra Bloom (2005) notes that survivors remember "the trauma in nonverbal, visual, auditory, kinesthetic, visceral, and affective modalities, but [are] not able to 'think' about it or process the experience in any way" (p. xvi). Survivors often will develop a freeze, flight, or fight response to trauma as a means of surviving. To continue to function in the world, trauma survivors would benefit from beginning to live in their bodies and slowly start to integrate thoughts and feelings as these relate to the trauma they have experienced.

Drama Therapy Defined

The use of drama therapy has proven to be quantitatively effective for individuals who have experienced trauma. Renee Emunah defined drama therapy as "the intentional and systematic use of drama/theatre processes to achieve psychological growth and change" (1994, p. 3). Through the use of embodiment-based therapy methods, such as drama therapy, trauma can safely be worked through to create cohesion, integration, and wholeness for individuals who often feel a sense of fragmentation.

The Importance of Aesthetic Distance with Trauma

Individuals, families, organizations, and communities can heal and thrive through the use of drama therapy methods which incorporate film and video. Performance provides a safe aesthetic distance, which assists trauma survivors with integrating painful feelings and experiences in a way that results in positive growth and change. Through the use of drama therapy and embodiment methods, both participants and those witnessing develop what Dr. Daniel Siegel (2010) terms "mindsight." Performers and observers of purposeful performance strengthen their middle prefrontal cortex, the area of the brain responsible for executive decision-making, problem-solving, emotional regulation, and self-understanding. Both performers and those witnessing a purposeful performance experience relief, catharsis, and healing. Judith Glass

(2006) explains "aesthetic distance," a term coined by Dr. Robert Landy, as a "therapeutic concept and touchstone for assessment of the effectiveness of treatment. Aesthetic distance is defined as the point at which the client can have access to his feelings and also maintain an observer stance" (p. 58).

Drama therapists assess the people they serve by observing whether they are overdistanced or underdistanced. Overdistance is when we are functioning in the world by overly relying on our thoughts and are removed from our feelings and our bodies. Underdistance is when we become overly emotional and limited in our ability to access our thoughts, reason, and rational mind.

In his book *The Couch and the Stage*, Landy (2007) references the work of Annette Streeck-Fisher and Bessel van der Kolk, who share six goals for treating trauma:

1   Safety
2   Stabilizing impulsive aggression against self and others
3   Affect regulation
4   Promoting mastery of experiences
5   Compensating for specific developmental deficits
6   Judiciously processing both the traumatic memories and trauma-related expectations.

The trauma-informed goals included below are from van der Kolk's work (Crenshaw, 2006; Streeck-Fischer & van der Kolk, 2000).

•   Developing an awareness of oneself and of the trauma
•   Learning to observe what is happening in the present and physically respond to current demands instead of re-creating the traumatic past behaviorally, emotionally, and biologically
•   Teaching self-soothing to cope with hyper-aroused physiological systems
•   Finding meaning; developing a positive orientation to the future.
                              (Streeck-Fischer & van der Kolk, 2000, p. 24)

Landy (2007) goes on to share how the role method, a drama therapy approach, is highly effective for trauma survivors because the container of taking on a fictional role creates a safe distance from the painful memory. Through role method and story, trauma survivors are able to regulate their affect and create what Landy terms a "cognitive bridge" between the fictional role and story and the trauma survivor's real-life experience (p. 224).

Role Theory is a drama therapy approach to treatment by the application of the role method. *Role theory* and *role method* are terms coined by Dr. Robert Landy and can be followed in eight steps:

1   Invoking the role.
2   Naming the role.
3   Playing out/working through the role.
4   Exploring alternative qualities in sub-roles.
5   Reflecting upon the role-play.
6   Relating the fictional role to everyday life.
7   Integrating roles to create a functional role system.
8   Social modeling: discovering ways that clients' behavior in a role affects others in their social environments.

According to van der Kolk (2014):

> Theater is about finding ways of telling the truth and conveying deep truths to your audience. This requires pushing through blockages to discover your own truth, exploring and examining your own internal experience so that it can emerge in your voice and on stage.
>
> (p. 337)

Bloom (2005) adds:

> Drama creates the opportunity for performative change, the creation of that "special force field"… that moves the human mind and the human nervous system.
>
> (p. xvii)

For trauma survivors, the use of embodiment, aesthetic distancing, purposeful performance, story, role, role-method, and the integration of the guide role supports healing and transformative change.

Embodiment is a drama therapy term and a tool individuals utilize to enact various roles' feelings and challenges by using their physical body as means of communication and self-expression. Embodiment drama therapy practices are especially valuable and effective for various reasons with individuals who have experienced trauma. First, by embodying our internal state, feelings, and obstacles, one can experience positive affect by externalizing one's inner experiences and thoughts. Second, embodiment as a tool for positive change and healing is effective for trauma survivors to communicate their painful experience without needing to be verbal. Third, embodiment also brings trauma survivors catharsis and an immediate way to discharge pain.

Aesthetic distance is a term coined by one of the pioneers of the drama therapy field, Robert Landy. "Aesthetic distancing" is a term used as a treatment goal for trauma survivors. Similar to being engrossed in a well-performed piece of theater, film, or television show, we are able to simultaneously reflect on the role, emerging issues, and overall piece and also feel with our emotions. The observers and performers involved in a purposeful piece experience catharsis and can both feel their emotions and reflect and cognitively process their experience.

> Any good work should be documented. Video seemed to be the best way to do that so that people could see it.
>
> (Campbell, 2020b, interview with Robert Landy)

Landy's first video-based approach emerged in the early 1980s when he served as a professor at New York University. He called his first approach the "extended dramatization." His three-step process for this approach is listed below.

Step 1. Sit in front of the monitor/camera for two minutes.
Step 2. Watch the video and comment on what you see. Ex: I see sadness, etc.
Step 3. Reflect on what you saw.

Landy always thought about the use of video and documenting even as he was building the field of drama therapy.

The use of video and film provides an additional tool for people who have experienced a trauma to self-regulate, gain insight, reach emotional catharsis, and develop new pathways for coping and problem-solving. Through the use of projection, role-play, embodiment, externalization, and the use of performance-based drama therapy, film, video, and playback theater, healing can occur along with bringing potentially painful stories and lived experiences to life in a safe way. There is healing in bringing trauma to light. Illuminating one's truth in a way where an individual feels deeply seen, heard, validated, and acknowledged breaks the silence and shame that often lingers around trauma. As trauma occurs in relationship, it heals in relationship. Film illuminates connection and healing when relationships are healthy, loving, and secure, but it also can lead individuals to become triggered and retraumatized in relationship.

Creating Educational and Therapeutic Impact using Trauma-Informed Drama Therapy in a Documentary Film: *Standing Tall*

Nearly 20 years ago as a young, aspiring drama therapist in graduate school studying drama therapy at New York University, I had the opportunity to learn from one of the pioneers in the field, Dr. Robert Landy. I recall sitting on a wooden floor, engrossed while watching the documentary film he worked on called *Standing Tall*. *Standing Tall* was filmed in 2001 shortly after the world watched as the World Trade Center towers crumbled. Landy met with a classroom of fourth-grade students who had witnessed the buildings collapse that unforgettable morning from their classroom window on September 11, 2001.

Dr. Landy, assisted by Damaris Webb (a teaching artist at City Lights Youth Theatre) and Christa Kirby (a drama therapy student), worked with the children using drama therapy approaches and purposeful performance as a way to support the students in healing by providing them a creative and safe outlet to express themselves and process the traumatic event they had observed.

Several weeks into the project, documentary film director Peggy Stern and her audio and camera team attended the drama therapy groups to document the work Landy and Webb were doing with the students. Stern and her team also went to the children's residences and interviewed them along with their families. Landy noted, "In their creative process they discovered that villains are as human as victims and heroes can be ordinary people, such as mothers." After the children's performance, Landy based the script for *Standing Tall* on the children's roles and stories that emerged during their work together.

The objectives for the *Standing Tall* project included the following:

1   To understand the human need to tell stories as a means of making sense of difficult, potentially traumatizing experiences
2   To understand the therapeutic value of role-playing, storytelling, and story dramatization
3   To understand the concept of aesthetic distance in transforming potential trauma in real life into safely contained forms of enactment
4   To extract a sense of meaning from the events of September 11, 2001, for children and adults.

(Landy, The Couch and the Stage, 2007)

The students participated in drama therapy techniques such as role theory, invoking the role, original storytelling, and therapeutic theater. The resulting film—*Standing Tall*—became a therapeutic and educational tool for working with trauma using drama therapy, story, role, and film.

The children role-played what the roles of hero, villain, and victim meant to them. In groups, the students were invited to create stories based on the theme of standing tall. Through role-play, metaphor, embodiment, story, and aesthetic distance, the students were able to reflect on their painful experience in a meaningful way.

Landy took the students' individual stories to create one collective narrative which was centered around the Island of Standing Tall. This performance was shared with the children's families and the school employees. Landy shared in an interview with me in April 2020 that the children from *Standing Tall* served as guides for the adults. After the children performed, they held a dialogue with the audience comprised of teachers, families, and friends. Landy noted that "for some adults, it was the first opportunity to speak and to release feelings about their experience of the terrorist attacks" (Landy, 2007, p. 224). Watching this powerful film in 2004 when I was a graduate student at New York University filled me with inspiration and hope as I embarked on the further stages of my drama therapy journey.

Close to 20 years after this film was made, Robert Landy shared his experience working on this powerful drama therapy film. Landy shared how the children's purposeful performance about a difficult experience, presented in a safely distanced manner, allowed them to create a safe space in which the audience of family, friends, and school staff could reflect, heal, and speak about their feelings related to the tragic event. The children also served as guides for the team of people who worked collaboratively on *Standing Tall*. In an interview, Landy noted how one of the students, also named Robert, often used comedy as a way to process, express, and heal. Landy shared how having young Robert in class and his use of comedy during the project deeply influenced, inspired, and informed Landy's own work and experience on that project.

Positive Educational and Therapeutic Outcomes

Students who participated in the *Standing Tall* theater program stated:

> "My whole world was dying."
> "If we didn't have the drama class, it would been different."
> "The drama class changed my life."
>
> (Campbell, 2020b)

Dr. Landy noted in our interview how much the acclaimed Academy Award winner and filmmaker Peggy Stern was positively impacted by her work on *Standing Tall*. The film seemingly catapulted her career, as she went on to work on films about various social issues and themes such as dyslexia, which she is reported to have struggled with.

As both a therapeutic and an educational tool, Landy explained that he showed *Standing Tall* across the globe and that many teachers referred to the manual that was created which included the use of theater-based approaches, incorporating these drama approaches into their curriculum.

Landy also noted that after sharing this film globally with thousands of viewers, adults began to share, for the first time, their own recollection of where they were in the world on September 11. Essentially, *Standing Tall* both was an educational tool for what trauma-informed drama therapy looks like and served as a therapeutic tool to address the world's collective trauma, creating space for healing to occur. Role, story, and purposeful performance are the safe containers in which to hold the trauma the children, their families, and the school were exposed to, along with the greater audience of people who viewed the film.

Creating Connections and Healing through Performance: The Therapeutic and Global Impact of the Witness Theatre

Founded in Israel in 2005 by Irit and Ezra Dagan, a married couple, the Witness Theatre pairs adolescents with survivors of the Holocaust, creating a space where stories of survival and loss are performed. The success of the Witness Theatre grew, such that a home was built for it in 2012 across the Atlantic Ocean by Selfhelp Community Services, one of the largest agencies assisting survivors in New York City (https://www.witnesstheaterthefilm.com/witness-theater).

In 2018, a documentary film titled *Witness Theater* was released (Rudavsky, 2018). The film depicted Holocaust survivors working in connection with adolescents who have a deep interest in hearing their stories. The creative process is led by a drama therapist and culminates in a meaningful performance. The performance includes projections of the survivors and memories of their past. This performance is shown to an audience and is simultaneously both livestreamed and filmed. Witness Theatre's performances are viewed globally and have positively impacted the survivors, adolescents, and those witnessing the film.

Outcomes

In a 2020 interview, trauma-informed drama therapist Jessica Asch noted that the group of adolescents and Holocaust survivors meet twice after the performance with the intention to both celebrate and reflect on the process (Campbell, 2020a). The layers of witnessing which occur during Witness Theatre performances and within the documentary bring forth important therapeutic objectives which include catharsis, validation, empathy, and being deeply seen and understood. Through purposeful performance and playing back the survivors' real stories, important connections were made which have a lasting impact on the adolescents and survivors involved and those who see the film.

Shine MSD and Camp Shine: A Therapeutic/Clinical, Research-Based, Educational, and Advocacy Tool

Shine MSD is a nonprofit organization founded in 2018 by two adolescents—Sawyer Garrity and Andrea Pena—after the tragic school shooting which occurred at Marjory Stoneman Douglas High School in Parkland, Florida on February 14 of that year. In 2020, an interview was conducted with Jessica Asch, a Licensed Creative Arts Therapist and Registered Drama Therapist who worked as the lead clinician at Camp Shine, the creative arts therapy program offered to survivors of the Parkland school shooting.

Asch shared that her work in 2018 using drama therapy and film within Camp Shine, a mere four months after the tragic event, focused on repairing the broken community and using the arts to connect and heal the divide resulting from the trauma it experienced. Her work with the students during 2019, the second year after the tragedy, focused on assessing their desire to live. Through video-based drama therapy work, students were able to step into their future selves and exhibit the hopefulness they possessed when considering their lives moving forward.

Videos of the students' dramatic enactments and spontaneous monologues were captured and immediately played back to be watched. Asch recalled students who role-played envisioning themselves going on to live happy and successful lives. The adolescents who participated in this drama therapy class role-played being an Olympic swimmer, a life-saving surgeon, a pop star, a movie director, and a computer programmer. Two participants selected the role of the average person—with a family, a pet, a home, a car, and a career—because of their desire for their lives to feel normal again.

Evidence-Based Research Outcomes

Hylton et al. (2019) conducted an evidence-based research study with the adolescents who participated in Camp Shine. Their article, titled "Improvements in Adolescent Mental Health and Positive Affect Using Creative Arts Therapy After a School Shooting: A Pilot Study" was written after surveying the participants. The authors concluded that for students in the Camp Shine drama therapy group, symptoms of PTSD, stress, anxiety, and depression significantly decreased, while positive affect increased in comparison to art therapy and music therapy interventions.

The Social Impact of Using Film and Theater to Raise Awareness and Advocate for Gun Reform

Level Forward is a theater production company which has connected with the nonprofit organization Shine MSD. Created by Abigail Disney and Adrienne Becker in 2018, Level Forward "develops, produces and finances high quality entertainment with Oscar- and Tony-winning producers." This company is unique in that its overall process includes a focus on social responsibility and thus creates a social impact both financially and by adding social value (https://www.levelforward.co/about).

Level Forward created an initiative called Gun Neutral "to offset the portrayal of guns on screens with a commitment to destroy ten firearms for every one that is featured in any of its productions" (Littleton, 2018). In addition to the reduction of illegal firearms, the Gun Neutral initiative connects with Level Forward to donate funds to arts-based programs located in communities impacted by gun violence. In the words of Level

Forward cofounder Adrienne Becker, "If you pair (storytelling) with the dialogue and the active advocacy then you have something really powerful" (Littleton, 2019).

Three Approaches to Drama Therapy: *An Educational Tool*

The film *Three Approaches to Drama Therapy*, made in 2004, is often used as an educational tool, covering the three main approaches known in drama therapy as Role Theory, Developmental Transformations, and Psychodrama (Siegel & Bryson, 2011) This film was made by Robert Landy in part within the Drama Therapy Department at New York University (Landy, 2004). I was present for this film's creative process, as at the time I was a second-year student in that department.

This film was modeled after the famous *Three Approaches to Psychotherapy* (Shostrom, 1965a, 1965b) and was successful in its ability to educate others about role theory, developmental transformations, and psychodrama. Robert Landy led the role theory portion of the film while working with a volunteer named Derek. David Read Johnson led the developmental transformations part of the film, and Nina Garcia led the psychodrama portion. What was not expected was the controversial nature of the use of developmental transformations with the main subject, Derek.

Landy shared how the film elicited strong feelings both within the drama therapy community and abroad when he did speaking engagements and attended conferences. Landy noted how some people were "horrified" by parts of the developmental portion shown between Dr. Johnson and Derek. In the film, Derek shares his adverse childhood experiences and recalls how his father was abusive toward him when he was a child. Within the participatory frameworks of role theory, psychodrama, and developmental transformation, Derek works through his trauma.

Through developmental transformations, Derek plays out evocative themes such as race, slavery, abuse, and power and control. With Johnson leading Derek in developmental transformations, Derek role-plays these difficult themes in a spontaneous manner.

When I interviewed Robert Landy, it was noted that Derek had been impacted by his involvement in the film and had subsequently gone "below the radar" for many years. The response has been mixed according to Landy, with half of the large numbers of people who have seen it finding it to be a valuable and educational tool. The other half find it difficult to watch and protest adamantly against the use of playing out the aforementioned themes with someone with a trauma background. Landy shared how one colleague walked out of a drama therapy conference, and also spoke out about having the film pulled from a major university's curriculum.

Since this film's release in 2005, the field of drama therapy has attracted many people of color and individuals from more diverse backgrounds and cultures than that of the White-centric drama therapy community that it had previously. Landy also shared that now more safeguards have been implemented when working with individuals using film and video, due to protecting confidentiality.

New York University's program director, Dr. Nisha Sajnani (2020), is incorporating film and video in her work by redoing a new version of *Three Approaches to Drama Therapy*. The future of the field of drama therapy depends on documenting and sharing our work by using film and video as an educational, therapeutic, research, and advocacy tool for social impact, change, and healing to occur in working with trauma.

References

Bloom, S. L. (2005). Foreword. In A. M. Weber & C. Haen (Eds.), *Clinical applications of drama therapy in child and adolescent treatment* (pp. xv–xviii). Brunner-Routledge.

Campbell, B. (2020a). Interview with Jessica Asch.

Campbell, B. (2020b). Interview with Robert Landy.

Crenshaw, D. (2006). Neuroscience and trauma treatment: Implications for creative arts therapists. In L. Carey (Ed.), *Expressive and creative arts methods for trauma survivors* (pp. 21–38). Jessica Kingsley.

Emunah, R. (1994). *Acting for real: Drama therapy process, technique, and performance*. Brunner/Mazel.

Glass, J. (2006). Working toward aesthetic distance: Drama therapy for adult victims of trauma. In L. Carey (Ed.), *Expressive and creative arts methods for trauma survivors* (pp. 57–71). Jessica Kingsley.

Hylton, E., Malley, A., & Ironson, G. (2019). Improvements in adolescent mental health and positive affect using creative arts therapy after a school shooting: A pilot study. *The Arts in Psychotherapy, 65*. doi: 10.1016/j.aip.2019.101586

Landy, R. J. (Director & Producer). (2004). *Three approaches to drama therapy*. [Documentary film]. 3 hours 47 minutes. Available from NYU Drama Therapy Program at nyudramatherapy@yahoo.com

Landy, R. J. (2007). *The couch and the stage: Integrating words and action in psychotherapy*. Jason Aronson.

Littleton, C. (2018, October 25). Level Forward sets Gun Neutral initiative for Killer Films' 'American Woman'. *Variety*. https://variety.com/2018/film/news/gun-neutral-level-forward-killer-films-american-woman-1202993976/

Littleton, C. (2019, October 9). Listen: Level Forward's Abigail Disney, Adrienne Becker on changing the industry, Bob Iger's paycheck. *Variety*. https://variety.com/2019/biz/news/abigail-disney-level-forward-adrienne-becker-oklahoma-1203365220/

Reneau, A. (2020, April). A trauma psychologist weighs in on the risks of 'motivational' pressure during quarantine. Upworthy. Retrieved from: https://www.upworthy.com/coronavirus-productivity-motivation-myths-dangers

Rudavsky, O. (Director). (2018). *Witness theater* [Documentary film]. https:// www.witnesstheaterthefilm.com/witness-theater

Shostrom, E. L. (Producer). (1965a). *Three approaches to psychotherapy* [Film]. Psychological Films.

Shostrom, E. L. (Producer). (1965b). *Three approaches to psychotherapy* [Transcript]. Psychological Films.

Siegel, D. J. 2010). *Mindsight: The new science of personal transformation.* Bantam Books.

Siegel, D. J., & Bryson, T. P. (2011). *The whole-brain child: 12 revolutionary strategies to nurture your child's developing mind.* Delacorte Press.

Stern, P. (Director & Producer). (2004). Standing tall [Film]. Fanlight Productions. www.fanlight.com

Streeck-Fischer, A., & van der Kolk, B. A. (2000). Down will come baby, cradle and all: Diagnostic and therapeutic implications of chronic trauma on child development. *Australian and New Zealand Journal of Psychiatry, 34*(6), 903– 918. doi: 10.1080/000486700265

van der Kolk, B. (2014). *The body keeps the score: Brain, mind, and body in the healing of trauma.* Penguin Random House. https://www.levelforward.co/about

8 The Wolfpack

Film as Therapy for the Soul

Joanna N. Dovalis

Psychotherapy provides a path to self-understanding as clients explore the relationship between the inner life and the outer world. *The Wolfpack* (Moselle, 2015) portrays a glimpse into the sheltered lives of a family on their journey of self-revealing and healing. James Hillman (1996) believed in the idea that people entered depth psychotherapy not only to seek symptom relief, or trace the origins of their traumatic wounding, but also to find an adequate biography that describes their singular lives in an emotionally intact way. In doing so, patients increase self-understanding and broaden their narrative as they embrace a bigger life. This active process frees one from being the victim of their personal life story to becoming the protagonist, supporting Jung's dictum that "we never get over anything, but we can grow out of it." The personality of the patient expands as a result of the healing that occurs not only in the transitional space between the therapist and the client—what Thomas Ogden (1994, p. 93) has described as the mysterious "analytic third"—but, more profoundly, in the transitional space between the ego and the Self. It is in this relational space that the ego no longer directs life choices, but surrenders its position of authority to the central archetype of the Self, the superordinate regulating center in the collective and personal unconscious, encompassing wholeness and potentiality. This process requires a firm ego. The *telos* (purpose) of the Self in the individuation journey is the hard psychological work of integration, which uses one's critical faculties (the four functions in Jungian typology) to unite the dark and light aspects of the psyche. In the film *The Wolfpack*, we witness how the development of an adequate biography aids the weaving together of the two realities in which we all live: the subjective world of the inner life and the imagination, and the outer world that compels confrontation with the other.

Film as the Mythopoetic World

Throughout this chapter, and consistent with a Jungian perspective, film and psychological, physical, and spiritual healing find common ground in the mythopoetic world. Ellenberger (1970) used the term *mythopoetic* to

DOI: 10.4324/9781315622507-11

describe an elemental function of the unconscious and its tendency to present itself to consciousness in the form of images that trend in the direction of archaic and archetypal motifs and images. Jung explained that these mythopoetic images have roots in the collective layer of the unconscious. The mythopoetic realm is a matrix that represents an intermediate space between the spiritual world and material reality. This "third" area is known as *psychic reality* or *imaginal reality*. In the realm of this deep stratum of the psyche, we perceive experience as spiritual. As Kalsched (2013) expresses in his book *Trauma and the Soul*, we live our actual lives "between the worlds" (p. 316). In our healthy selves, we are "citizens of two realms" (p. 316). It is within these spaces that we can consciously relate to the emotional and archetypal patterns of our birth and fate cards and influence the direction of our destiny. By living our real nature within a vital and animated core self, we are enabled to express life more creatively.

As psychotherapists, we traditionally define trauma in the context of a relational field. We inquire about the personal history of the patient and review their present life experiences and suffering along with their dreamwork to guide therapy toward understanding and healing. Early trauma often occurs in the earliest attachment between the child and his or her primary caretaker. Trauma forecloses on transitional space as a result of overwhelming experiences that the child is unable to metabolize, which leads to those experiences being repressed into the unconscious. James Grotstein (2000) suggests that trauma is about encountering the world before the baby has the chance to create it. However, Neville Symington (1993) emphasizes that trauma experienced in childhood is not the crucial factor in the development of primitive defenses; instead, it is the individual's *response* to the trauma that matters most.

In the film *Wolfpack*, the group of brothers experiences trauma starting in their early years, although their mother appears to be completely devoted and emotionally available to them. The boys' trauma is not about their relationship with their primary caretaker, but with the other—their father—and consequently the outer world, they have been deprived of knowing. Their inner world of attachment appears to be well in place, but for the sake of their emotional and social development, they must meet the outer world.

Into the Outer World

The Wolfpack begins with a stunning synchronistic event in the lives of the six Angulo brothers, during which the director Crystal Moselle finds them escaping the confines of their imprisoning childhood home. This synchronous event reveals a mysterious sense of the boys' inner world colliding with the outer world: from the life in which they were living to the life to which they are escaping. This profound moment in time transcends the otherwise clear boundary between self and other. The beginning scenes exemplify Jung's belief that dreams and synchronicities emerge from an active intelligence in the unconscious. The individual charges the world that challenges himself to take up a very difficult and rewarding contest, as if reenacting the defeat of the Titan god Saturn, who ate all his progeny, save one—Zeus—who overthrew him. This survival not only supplants old hierarchies but realizes, by the very act of overturning, the boys' desire to break through to a broader perspective and ultimate experiences of self-discovery, liberation, authentic suffering, and acceptance. It is not only a part of great stories passed over oceans and through time. It is, at the center, a story about seeking and eventually realizing one's soul concerning others and the Other. Moreover, as the aptly and magically named Crystal supposes, if not by design, a great deal more is going on than watching six brothers ape movie characters to avoid being Saturn's next snack. For the Angulo brothers, their remarkable relationship to the world of film proves to be the window to the external world: that world which, as they self-report, has saved them.

Kalsched's (2013) work on trauma emphasizes that "often the early story of the trauma survivor is a mythological story before it is personal one" (p. 5), supporting Jung's discovery of the collective unconscious and the archetypal reservoir of the ancient psyche which provides a matrix of imagery that serves as an in-depth resource for the living soul. Kalsched (2010) quotes the analyst Trousdale, who observes that "trauma produces a heightened drama of heroes and victims whose more ordinary story is waiting to be told" (p. 131). It landed on Otto Rank in his book on the *Myths of the Birth of the Hero* (2015), which identifies five essential constituents of a myth. The biography of *The Wolfpack* follows this mythological order:

1 The infant is born to noble or divine parents or is the issue of a deity and an early maiden, sometimes a virgin. Difficulties such as prolonged barrenness in the parents or depression in the community precede his origin.
2 The "extraordinary signs and prophecies" attending the pregnancy or the infant's birth arouse the anxiety of the ruling king or of the infant's father, who sets out to kill or banish him.
3 The infant is "exposed" to die, or is surrounded by the sea in a basket, or is sent away or escapes owing to the intervention of benevolent forces that intervene. Sometimes this is the infant's mother. Sometimes miraculous warnings come through dreams.
4 The infant is rescued—sometimes by animals, a humble woman, or a fisherman—and brought up in another land.
5 The hero, now a youth, returns to overthrow the father and/or renew the community through his leadership.

The mythological story of Zeus and his child-devouring father, Chronos, is embedded in the personal lives of the *Wolfpack* boys. The myth describes children who are born between two worlds: one human, the other divine. The powers of an egoistic, patriarchal authority threatens their lives. The myth resolves when Zeus transcends his fate by acquiring a sense of power from non-ordinary means. Often in myths, the transcendent vehicle comes in the form of oracles or dreams whereby one is able to circumvent one's fate at birth and, as a result, live out his or her true nature and destiny. As a modern myth, the *Wolfpack* boys' sense of aliveness is preserved by the mythopoetic world of film and saved by the successful synchronous event during which they run into the producer: a being who is pivotal in changing the boys' destiny. Thus, it is helpful to view the film as it devours its 85 minutes by marking certain places in its chronology during which the eyes truly become windows to the soul. This will not stake a claim for the greatness of this particular film, but to show how old wine ever makes its way into new bottles. On the surface, it replays the necessary discard of an old system for a new one, where growth can occur in this household. Indeed, the six brothers, and ultimately their mother, as subjects in this alleged documentary, are aware that they not only manifest "evident facts" about the strange domestic arrangement in which they find themselves but also comment on it, act on it, and, ultimately, in some hip meta-movie magic, become more themselves as they meet the Other.

The backstory is simple enough. On a wintry morning on Manhattan's Lower East Side, the mythical melting pot of a multiethnic and multidimensional America, the producer encountered six brothers on the sidewalk. All were dressed in black, each imitating the look of characters in the film *Junkyard Dog* (Bass, 2010), one of the future lupines' favorites. Moselle, a film-schooled producer in the making, was not only attracted to their Hindu names (derived from Sanskrit), or their homeschooling, or their waist-length hair. She also shared a love of movies with these engaging yet outré kids. They were children of the housing projects. However, unlike the latchkey wanderers of their caste, these boys had not been allowed to venture into the city but grew up in the confines of a large apartment. There they existed, locked in by their father and homeschooled by their certified mother. A collection of DVDs and VHS tapes that cut a big swath through Hollywood tinsel and tradition largely comprised the boys' library. The Wolfpack emerged from this encounter, after the moment the sons chose not to become snacks for the jealous patriarchal god, Oscar.

The boys' father, Oscar Angulois, is absent throughout the first half of the film, which serves as a symbolic gesture by the director, as it represents how Oscar had been emotionally absent throughout his sons' development. It is the father's role, as the masculine parent, to prepare his children for the external world. Limits, boundaries, and rules must be taught to guide the children into independence to meet the demands of the conditional outside world. In this regard, Oscar has failed his sons. He possesses the only key to the door, physically and emotionally controlling the boys' separation process.

It is also important to note that the boys' only sister is also absent from the narrative of the entire film. This omission also appears to be intentional by the director, representing a lone wounded feminine, something the daughter is unconsciously holding for her mother. Although the children have a devoted mother who freely gives her family her full attention and unconditional love, she has unconsciously colluded with her husband in his distorted idea of protection. It is a witty and devastating setup. Oscar will be shown to be a dupe of his inflated, charismatic narcissism and fecklessness.

Other key points in the backstory might slip past us. For one, the producer appears in some scenes in the pack's apartment. Another is that the precipitate event—in which a child sets forth as done by ancient heroes—occurs prior to the start of the film. That crucial event, therefore, appears as de facto—almost routine—in the course of the narrative. Much of the first 25 minutes onscreen establishes the curious and surreal household ordained by Oscar, an exotic father who imagines himself as the semen bearer of a race of Krishna gods, who do his bidding in the name of minimal contact with the immediate outside world. This presentation further depicts the powerful influence of movies in creating the worldview through which the boys live and ultimately begin to throw off the old regime. Oscar is withheld from view, like the other monsters in the Anglo Saxon *Beowulf*, so as to allow the auditor's febrile imaginations to concoct a private terror. However, we will arrive at the place this terror abates soon enough.

The film opens with a string of inchoate and mildly jarring images and sounds as if we have stumbled into an edit session. These combine to create a greater sense of dislocation into which brief and coherent comments and business by the family create an alternative sense of psychological order based on superheroes and a library of 5,000 movies. In this mélange of establishing shots and bits of dialogue, three seem to stand out in particular. The confinement makes film dialogue the shielding wall of the old epic and familiar space operas, like *Star Wars*. Indeed, the movies provide both the lingua franca and the cornerstone of identity for the pack of boys. Unlike Alice, who falls into the underworld in pursuit of the white rabbit, these boys were raised on the other side of the looking glass. So in the opening montage—itself very disorienting—the running descent down steel stairs suggests not only a desperate escape, at once reminiscent of disaster movies, but also a descent from luminous illusions of film surfaces and dreams into the reality beneath. That this image is repeated suggests that Moselle wants to make sure her point is well taken.

The first of these flashpoints involves the pack waving their "Top 100 all-time movies" list. Their unanimous picks for top positions are the first two parts of *The Godfather* (Coppola, 1972/1974), another romp through the demands of power hierarchies and patriarchs. Their unanimous vote reflects the power of the collective in their small tribe. The list also appears to contain *Citizen Kane, Casablanca,* one of the *Batman* movies, and *Superfly*—this last providing a bit of urban racial mimicry in good fun. The list signifies that order of sorts exists in this apartment. This pack of boys has viewed plenty of movies and has rated them, just like other people in the city of Manhattan. The boys' collective consensus reflects the power of sibling relationships. They have been fortunate to have each other during their confinement, and their sheer number has prepared them for the social interactions of a larger world that they soon will meet.

The second powerful sequence is a talking head interview with the boy's mother, Susan. She asserts with some pride how she has been certified for homeschooling by the City's Kafka-esque educational establishment and that after seven pregnancies her body gave up the quest for producing ten little deities, sired by Oscar. The number ten is a symbolic representation of Oscar's distorted spiritual quest for wholeness, but his master plan has been aborted by the wisdom of the unconscious feminine—the mother's body. Susan further relates that she had left the Midwest to adventure in the Andes, thus explaining how she met and fell for Oscar, a tour guide in Peru. Her one-sided need to leave the security and stability of the status quo represented by Midwestern values swung to its opposite compensatory side for adventure, landing her in the shadows of the underworld. The mother's moon-eyed and straightforward tone is chilling. She may be drinking Oscar's Kool-Aid, but she seems not to mind. Susan and her children live in the unconscious symbiotic realm of the Great Mother, a state of participation mystique in great need of separation.

A third sequence of the film shows the boys exhibiting their creative gifts of improvisation and creation of their cardboard set and costume design, usually constructed from readily available materials like cereal packages. Had these children been dimwitted and sullen, this would be a slasher movie. But they are insouciant and raucous, and although one wolf admits to total ignorance about "talking to girls," there is a distinct impression that the boys' enforced isolation has not dumbed them to a false sense of reality. Indeed, in passing, they remark about a passion for reading to supplement the over-amped cinematic upon which they feed. The ironic truth may be that movies alone had not saved them from the boredom of living such a small life; by being homeschooled, they were also protected from the more negative influences of life outside their front door. Living in this confined space and with the constant pressure of suffering, they had to rely on their creative instincts.

At about 25 minutes into the film, the oldest brother, who is 15 years old and well into adolescent development, recalls that one day when

Oscar was out shopping, he decided to go outside himself. Here is the hero of the family system, the knight setting forth into the dark wood of banks, drugstores, and grocery markets. Of course, not knowing this world, he left the apartment in disguise, dressed in black and wearing a facemask. "Someone called the cops," he recalls on screen. He was returned home, handcuffed, to nary a rebuke. The attire worn in going out is a movie costume. Manhattanites are accustomed to seeing weird stuff routinely, but some tawny young man in quasi SWAT dress serves to remind viewers that the boy, not the people fondling kale, is the Other. As might be expected, he ended up in an inpatient psychiatric hospital where he met regularly with a therapist. At this point, the world of these wolves has permanently shifted on its axis: the brother eventually moves out of the family home. This event epitomizes the toppled apple cart of a trauma initiating the separation process from his original family and independence. Ironically, the mother made a big deal in her interview about socialization: here, the errant Parsifal gets a first lesson in what has been missed in an illusory film world.

The three critical nodes in the next part of *The Wolfpack* are a trip to a real NYC movie house, the appearance of Oscar, and a trip to the beach at Coney Island. The movie's excursion is touching. The boys are all dressed up as they seek their symbolic confirmation; the relationship between their inner world and the external world has commenced. It must have been startling to view their celluloid habitat in the broader confines of the *temenos*, the sacred space of a movie emporium, what Raymond Chandler in an entirely different context called "a palimpsest brought out by ultraviolet light in a dark room." The stories contained in the pack collectively and personally crash upon the shore of another world. The palimpsest exists below the special effects, in shared memory and the unconscious.

The third episode takes us by subway and elevated train over the bridge to Coney Island and the southeastern-facing waters of the Atlantic Ocean. The bridge and train ride possess magic, the transitional space in which dangers are overcome, and, of course, psychological and physical movement from point A to point B occurs. What finer image of the underside of the persona exists? It is a beautiful scene. The seashore on which they frolic is likened to the transitional space in the mythopoetic realm. Between water and land, a union of opposites is occurring, creating a transcendent "third" space of integration. According to Winnicott (1971), transitional space is the space through which the child makes the crucial transition from omnipotence to the reality principle. Living in the mythopoetic space of film has undoubtedly kept the brothers' sense of aliveness well intact, yet they must abandon their identification with their roles as superheroes. Their active engagement and omnipotent feelings toward these mythical figures have protected them against feelings of profound powerlessness, a defense they have needed to survive their father's oppression. Psychologically, the oceanic experience is no longer a symbol of living in the unconscious waters with mother but is now a place of separation where they may touch the borderland depths and scope with the Other in themselves, as well as the Other on the outside.

In the final third of the film, the outer world intrudes as we learn that a neighbor had reported the household for its collection of sinister armaments. A SWAT team assault on the family ensues, resulting in everyone being handcuffed, including the young boys and their mother. Of course, the weapons are only movie-inspired props made of cardboard and duct tape. The world of the "Great Out There" has broken Oscar's spell with impunity and ruthless efficiency. The appearance of Oscar in his Panama straw hat makes him look like a worker on a coffee plantation. However, the real denigration of Oscar, once so feared and remote, is that though he speaks passable English, he is subtitled. The hilarious effect supposes that Oscar's defensive and entitled rationales for not working are the source of the outré in the household. He is like Frank Morgan behind the curtain, suddenly exposed as in the *Wizard of Oz*.

The next two high points include the reconnection of the children's mother with her 88-year-old mother, who have been estranged for half a century. We do not learn the dynamics behind this long separation, but it is clear some healing is about to occur. On a psychological level, we can only imagine that Susan has replicated an earlier trauma from her original family history and that the violent confrontation with outer reality has thrown her forward into the present. Something in her unconscious has been awoken, allowing her the imperative betrayal to her husband's pathology and the patriarchal order she had been organizing around, and permitting her to reconnect with the mother she says she thinks about every day. A union of a deeper feminine is occurring. She has returned to the source of her pain, something Jung emphasized when he suggested we must return to the *prima materia* in order to individuate.

The most magical scene in the film is a trip to the country. In an apple orchard, one of the boys tells his mom, "This is the best apple I ever had." Here is the fall in the Book of Genesis but in reverse, where the old prohibition and forbidden fruit become the image that supports integration with the larger world. The scene is a model of the sweet joy we feel when experiencing our own separateness and individuality. Yet the last scene just as quickly dumps us down the chute of despair. From the edifying pastoral detour, we see one boy, in his grocery-made fright mask, reminiscent of primitive masks most people see only in museums, with a long, slow-motion scream. This scene haunts us by reminding us that not all trauma survivors recover.

Confronting the Other entails the hard work of individuation, something Oscar was unable to do in his patriarchal role. Leaving the secure, if proscriptive, castle of the wounded anti-father would not be a day trip to Coney Island. Instead, making sense of their history, the Wolfpack boys must navigate the pixels and prisms of what seems to matter in a cinematic *Weltanschauung*. All we need is the Queen of Hearts, Alice's courage and curiosity, and a stubborn hold on a sense of wonder. Such stories are healing because they express the life journey, albeit in dramatic form, and the compensatory processes in the collective unconscious that work to balance one-sidedness: the sickness and the constant deviations of human consciousness.

References

Bass, K. (Writer & Director). (2010). *Junkyard dog* [Film]. Bass Entertainment.

Coppola, F. F. (Director). (1972/1974). *The godfather* [Film]. Paramount.

Ellenberger, H. F. (1970). *The discovery of the unconscious: The history and evolution of dynamic psychiatry*. Basic Books.

Grotstein, J. S. (2000). *Who is the dreamer, who dreams the dream? A study of psychic presences*. Routledge.

Hillman, J. (1996). *The soul's code: In search of character and calling*. Warner Books.

Kalsched, D. (2010). *Defenses in dreams: Clinical reflections on the multiplicity necessary for survival in pieces*. Paper presented at the *XVIIIth IAAP (International Association for Analytical Psychology) Congress*, Montreal, Canada, August 22–27, 2010.

Kalsched, D. (2013). *Trauma and the soul: A psycho-spiritual approach to human development and its interruption*. Routledge.

Moselle, C. (Director). (2015). *The wolfpack* [Film]. Magnolia.

Ogden, T. H. (1994). The analytic third: Working with intersubjective clinical facts. *The International Journal of Psychoanalysis, 75*(1), 3–19.

Rank, O. (2015). *The myth of the birth of the hero: A psychological interpretation of myth*. G. C. Richter & E. J. Lieberman (Trans.). (orig. pub. 1909). Johns Hopkins University Press.

Symington, N. (1993). *Narcissism: A new theory*. H. Karnac.

Winnicott, D. W. (1971). *Playing and reality*. Penguin.

9 Video Storytelling

The Influence of Video and How It Can Heal

Nancy Mramor Kajuth

Introduction

Visual media has the power to make you laugh, cry, hit the person next to you, get motivated, forgive, or judge yourself. Viewing visual media can change one's world. Research has proven over the past 50 years of movies and TV that the overt and covert messages of the media shape children through social learning, influence adults into buying things to make their lives better, and indirectly tell one who *should* be in their life (Mramor Kajuth, 2015).

Enter the element of psychotherapy. A therapy session always feels like a blank canvas when it begins. The aspects and strengths of the client, along with the tools and gifts of the therapist, combine to create an artwork of healing in unpredicted and fulfilling ways. However, what happens when visual media and therapy come together?

As a psychologist and producer for PBS-TV, creating a window into the world and the mind for viewers was a rewarding task. The production of psychology segments for an evening news show brought the elements of understanding the self and how we become who we are to the screen. Topics ranged from following a group of men from different walks of life who came together at the Warhol Museum to create art installations together, to the benefits of spending an afternoon at the Phipps Conservatory surrounded by plants, flowers, and butterflies. The outcome was always a piece of visual media art that expanded the experience of the viewer, offering the opportunity for personal growth and self-understanding. It was a lot like "psychology for everyman" without the heaviness of drama, but with an option to grow if it was to the viewer's liking.

Traditional media, however, is a more powerful influence in one's life; producers influence one's beliefs and behaviors by the ways that they carefully craft programming. The methods of influence in media production include elements of hypnosis that are highly effective in creating either false, hypnotic beliefs or positive beliefs that support one's authentic life.

DOI: 10.4324/9781315622507-12

The earliest studies on how we are affected by media sprung from a desire to determine if violent TV viewing is related to follow-up violent behavior in the viewer. It was proven to have an effect, and even today, there is an international awareness of the effects of televised violence. A study of German adolescents who were tested over two years looked at media violence use and aggressive behavior. Variables were carefully controlled, and media violence use was a significant predictor of both self-reported and teacher-reported aggression. No powerful effects were noted for nonviolent media, so it is not media viewing in itself that is the cause. High-violent media users also had lower empathy scores on test measures (Krahé et al., 2012). The evidence of aggression related to violent media viewing and a lack of empathy are consistent over time with many studies validating these effects.

However, on a positive note, video viewing can also have powerful healing outcomes. In the movie *The Upside of Anger* (2005) with Joan Allen and Kevin Costner, writer and director Mike Binder creatively illustrated the ways that anger can influence beliefs, human behavior, and relationships. The two and a half hours go by quickly as one observes and identifies with the characters. The assumptions are that one becomes the rules by which one lives, and if they are false, they can rob one of years of one's life. The painful effects of anger seem to break wide open upon learning that one's perceptions are one's reality.

The therapeutic effect of viewing this movie is that as one watches, identifies with the characters, and observes the lessons that they learn, one is learning them, too. One may always remember them, and one may tell others about them or even apply the lessons in their own life when an opportunity provides, but once viewed they are never the same (Mramor Kajuth, 2015).

By viewing consciously and learning the tools of the producer, a client can achieve the same result by producing their own life stories. The change that occurs is that media becomes a way to awaken rather than to be hypnotically put to sleep. Also, whether someone is behind the camera or in the audience, one can be the producer, director, and star in one's own life.

The role of the producer behind the scenes in the creation of the visual media can be a force for change and self-awareness. On February 28, 2016, the 88th Academy Awards were held to acknowledge films that made a difference. The award for best animated film went to Pete Docter and Jonas Rivera for their production of *Inside Out*, a film that showed kids that growing up isn't always easy. The movie asks the question, "Ever wonder why we feel the way we do?" examining emotions such as joy, anger, sadness, fear, and disgust, with full acknowledgment that sadness is a part of life. (Docter, 2015).

In accepting the award, Pete Docter admitted that the movie was born from parents watching kids grow up. He tells kids that "Some days you will feel angry, sad, scared, but make stuff, make films, draw, write." And he is right. Allowing feelings to flow through the arts has powerful effects.

Individual Influences in Media Viewing

Whether it is someone's personal life, a therapeutic process, health, career, or family, one is influenced by what one watches, and it shapes who they become (Bandura, 1997). Issues in one's personal life, and the ability to follow one's dreams and even one's appearance, are shaped by one's family, especially one's parents, mentors, and the media. The media especially can and should be used in a constructive way to influence whom one becomes. But the fact is that it is not always the case; media viewing can have a negative effect if one is not careful (Neubert, 2009). Glenn Sparks, professor of communications at Purdue University, found that people who watch forensic and crime dramas are more likely than non-viewers to have a distorted view of the criminal justice system and that they are likely to overestimate the frequency of crime (Neubert, 2009). Susan Sarapin, who researched with Sparks, reported that heavy users of TV crime estimated more than twice as many real-world murders than those who did not view massive crime shows. Their study sparked a discussion of "mean world syndrome," according to Sparks; people who start to think of the world as a scary place may develop feelings of being victimized (Neubert, 2009).

Because crime dramas are one of the most popular genres for media viewers, the effect of viewing violence is highly pertinent. Albert Bandura's early studies showed that whenever we witness aggression, it can change our behavior. However, TV violence may not be necessary for viewer satisfaction. Reports at Indiana University showed episodes of *24 Hours, The Sopranos*, and other crime shows with the violent scenes cut out and with them included. The test subjects reported that they enjoyed the shows with the violence removed significantly more than the individuals who saw the original versions (*IU News Room*, 2013).

Such a medium also has the power to change one for the positive good. The author was inspired to research the healing aspects of video viewing after making appearances on TV and radio. The discovery of the far-reaching capabilities of the media to disseminate information about psychology as a teaching tool spurred the project. With the support of a grant from a local college, research was conducted to discover if there were effects of viewing a televised curriculum of stress management with children. There were significantly less observed stress symptoms in the children, on observational measures completed by their teachers, following the treatment (Mramor, 1990). The curriculum was packaged and released worldwide following the completion of the study.

The next experience with healing video occurred following my recovery from leukemia in 2000, when the medical team joined in the creation of a DVD on *Hypnosis for Healing*. The words and images are designed to open the experience of the viewer to the possibility of healing. The University of Pittsburgh Medical Center Foundation at Shadyside Hospital funded the project, allowing for the completion of a tool for wellness in general, but especially for cancer patients. Their reports of the benefits include feelings of great calmness, renewed hope, and optimism following viewing.

Dr. Josh Cohen et al. (2015) proposes creating and viewing media can have a positive effect when the material is personal. When used creatively, the tools of media can be used purposefully to create healing and new beliefs. The creation of the entire production is an experience in healing. As soon as one starts to imagine one's production, they begin to visualize their *process of healing*, and the brain begins the healing process. Then, seeing the self the way one wants *their outcome* works further to convince the brain.

This philosophy is one that we share; the result was the release of the book, *Get Reel: Produce Your Own Life* in 2015. "Getting reel" means that anybody can control their viewing experience and viewing choices by becoming a savvy, conscious viewer of media. It is critical to developing such skills because social learning from movies and TV is an important part of who you become.

Changing Times and Media

The times change what we view, and we change the times by what we view. Social, financial, political, and environmental forces in the world influence what producers create to reflect the times. We also change in our own lives and influence what producers notice about us. In turn, we shape what they will produce.

In *Get Reel*, one learns how one is influenced and how they influence media in their relationships, politics, spending, spiritual beliefs, family dynamics, and self-esteem by media.

- Self-esteem is a critically important area not only because of the perfect images seen on TV but because of the subliminal messages that we must attain specific ways of looking and being in order to be happy.
- *Relationships* "as seen on TV" show us that love has to be either problematic or perfect, neither of which is accurate. While they make for interesting programming, when someone absorbs either of these beliefs, one is doomed in love. Viewers can even develop perceived close relationships with media figures viewed on TV. The level of satisfaction and amount of investment they make in the character are predictors of commitment to the character. Repeated exposures and the length of the encounters with the character may develop a sense of shared experiences (Branch et al., 2013).

- Heavier exposure to romantically themed movies is more closely associated with the belief that "Love finds a way." More substantial exposure to reality marriage-themed shows resulted in stronger beliefs of "Idealization" and "Love finds a way." Ninety-four percent of those surveyed indicated that they looked to movies for examples of romantic love, while only one-third looked to their mothers (Lippman et al., 2014). Media is thus an essential source of information about love.

- There is a spin on *politics* from the first time that information is presented. The stories that will get airtime are chosen, as are the details of the stories that are told. The commentaries are selected, and the viewer comments are picked from a large pool of different views. Whenever someone watches politics, one should use their finest conscious viewing skills to make their own decisions.

- Media-influenced values about money vary among cultures. Joseph Heinrich et al. (2010) played "The Ultimatum Game" to study how various cultures spend and perceive money.

- A *Journal of Media and Religion* study (Bobkowski, 2009) showed that religious productions depict spiritual beliefs and practices that influence viewers' spiritual beliefs. We know that religious teens prefer less mature entertainment. Moreover, spirituality explained 27 percent of the differences in happiness among children.

- As family dynamics change in media, they then adapt to the real family and vice versa. The show *The Middle*, reviewed by some critics as the best new comedy of 2009–2010, depicts a real middle-class family with challenges and hurdles to overcome. (Heline, & Heiser, 2009–2018). They deviate from the perfect images we saw in the 1950s and 1960s when *The Donna Reed Show, Father Knows Best*, and *Ozzie and Harriet* reflected the baby-boomer images of perfect families (Mramor Kajuth, 2015).

The Dynamics of Influence

The ways that Hollywood producers use to entertain, keep one viewing, and change how one thinks often come from modern hypnosis (Erickson, 1983). The following hypnotic methods, commonly used in entertaining productions, can be used positively in video-based therapy.

Anchoring is the act of repeating a message over and over until it is associated with the outcome that one desires. For example, using the same music behind scenes that include a positive message, reinforcing the message with smiling people having fun, attaching wealth, luxury, sex, or babies to stories where the association is not automatic are uses of anchoring. It is used most often in advertising but is an element of all influential documentaries. A positive message attached to film/video-based therapy, when repeated several times, will have therapeutic value.

Another method of influence is called *pattern interruption*. It is often used to surprise the viewer and keep them viewing. Someone thought the guy who killed Aunt Martha was the guy at the newsstand, and it turned out that the murderer was hiding behind the lilac bush. Changing course in a production shifts the thinking from what was to what is now or can be. A film/video-based therapeutic production that includes changes regarding the way the author felt before and after addressing a condition or trauma utilizes *pattern interruption* to promote healing when conducted by licensed professionals in the mental health industry.

Curiosity is also critical to conscious viewing. What is the message? What caused the crisis and what are the possible solutions? Curiosity precedes learning and is a critical feeling to evoke to keep a viewer engaged and to make the work compelling.

The use of these tools enhances viewer awareness, creates a new reality, and evokes a sense of completion. A sense of completion occurred after the most popular mini-series in public television history—*Downton Abbey*—ended, and all the loose ends were nicely sewn up. The same neat endings do not occur in real life, but an individual's ending is theirs alone, produced, created, and directed for their self-expression. Perhaps the healing cause is a group one, which means not having to go it alone. Joining with others in creating healing self-expression is another way that the art of video therapy can heal.

What Do We Know that Can Directly Influence Video Therapy?

Children are especially influenced by Bandura's concepts of social learning. Dr. Josh Cohen et al. (2015) discuss how children increasingly use the Internet and technology to address stress resulting from the death of a loved one, due to ease and availability. Their familiarity with technology makes them feel comfortable there, even if they are not fully aware of safety issues related to technology. Several points bear noting relative to the use of therapeutic video production.

- In a recent pilot study, therapeutic filmmaking activities, when added to counseling services at a university, resulted in reports of increased self-mastery and changes in perspective by participants (Johnson & Alderson, 2008).
- One interesting element of the process is that one becomes both the observer and the observed in cases when the video includes the self or a projected image that represents the self. The importance of the video multiplies overuse of simple cinema-therapy or viewing a therapeutic movie, such as the one noted earlier regarding *The Upside of Anger*.
- Children exposed to domestic violence often experience PTSD. Without treatment, those children experience a greater likelihood of suicide, substance abuse, depression, and victimization (Becker et al.,

2010). Digital storytelling overrides the difficulties that they may confront with verbalizing or expressing their emotions about their experiences. It also provides an opportunity for some closure by creating a conclusion to the story.

- Viewers of videos used to increase social wellness reported feeling that it was okay to discuss mental illness, that there was healing in the discussion, and even got other family members talking about it more.
- Veterans who avoided traditional therapy due to stigma and avoidance were able to use a narrative approach in a specific and intentional way that can make the memories more manageable.

Dr. Josh Cohen has been using Film/Video-Based Therapy (FVBT) to create and study the process of the therapeutic value of video and filmmaking for healing of the self and the community with licensed professionals in mental health. Therapeutic film production has many of the qualities found in traditional media that have been used in therapy for their healing possibilities. Therapists who have used video FVBT stated that the process heals through expression of the client's story. It moves material from the abstract unconscious into a "constructive storytelling event." The goal of making video to heal the self encompasses the theory of depth psychology because it aims toward the goals of integration and wholeness.

This type of storytelling is a process used by a person trained in therapeutic techniques and narrative storytelling to create an opportunity for both individuals and groups to release their story through a fun and therapeutic process. The entire process creates an environment in which clients can tell their stories through the merging of conscious logic and unconscious elements of the psyche, says Dr. Cohen. Based on my experience with production and editing for PBS, this belief is shared about elements of a video-based story. Anything that seems related to the topic is captured on film, and the individual elements that make up the story are gathered later. Then, some details of the larger story are chosen to be a part of the final production during editing, while others are not. Elements not chosen are those that are not considered as relevant or important to the telling of the story. The pieces of the story can be chosen and presented in an order that is either sequential in time or told through a series of current events and flashbacks that explain the importance of the event in real time. The process is one of integration of the parts into a meaningful whole, and while the decision-making process is a professional and personal one in the mainstream media, for the client it is deeply personal and therapeutic.

In FVBT, the editing process is similar to the process of psychotherapy in that the whole story is generally told, at first through conscious memories. Then, as those elements emerge, they often bring with them some unconscious elements that are attached to those conscious elements of awareness. The treatment modality of Eye Movement Desensitization and Reprocessing (EMDR), which is used to address trauma, is especially effective at bringing the less conscious thoughts to the surface. In FVBT, the client goes through the process of remembering and capturing in a video format those elements that best tell the personal story or the story of the larger issue. There is preparation and planning, shooting, and editing. Moreover, the final product is then refined through background narrative, picture, and sound editing. While the goal of traditional video production is for distribution, the goals of FVBT vary from client to client. For example, FVBT is especially relevant to Aboriginal clients, who face a number of barriers in traditional treatment due to the cultural values of therapists who do not understand the traumas which they have experienced or their cultural differences (Agius & Hamer, 2003).

Ancient Futures, a text penned by Helena Norberg-Hodge, was written during many years inside the indigenous culture of the gentle and pristine Ladakh culture in the Himalayan region of India near Tibet. The Westernization of the previously self-reliant people brought changes that created environmental, social, and mental health breakdown. Also, the media was partly responsible for the breakdown (Norberg-Hodge, 2009).

Radio and TV have replaced the need to sit around the fire and tell stories. Telling one's own stories and singing one's own songs is a self-conscious exercise; while the tribe used to compare themselves to one another, they are now comparing their efforts to the ones they see and hear on the screen. A world where everyone is glamorous and clean with fast cars, microwave ovens, and macho heroes has influenced the self-esteem of the culture, where people compare their lives to the illusions of perfection they see in the media.

Before the Westernization of their culture, the Ladakhis were happy, content, frugal, and self-reliant despite the harsh weather and the lack of modern conveniences. Now they are experiencing the culture shock of a rapidly changing world that is generating passivity and insecurity. Their definition of self-worth has changed due to shame that has been engendered by Western films about cowboys and Indians that make the Indian cultures look primitive. Perhaps a part of the cure is similar to the problem. Self-produced documentaries, along with a slower, more integrated style of globalization, could be elements of a solution.

Get Reel: Produce Your Own Life illustrates how the media affects the culture, for better and for worse. The impact of media on relationships, spending, happiness, health, family, self-esteem, and—most importantly— on ways of thinking and perceptions about the self, determines what one believes it takes to be happy. When viewing consciously, one pays attention to the messages that are sent, and viewing becomes an experience that strengthens the viewer in ways that match the authentic self.

An international study may lead us to a global understanding of the possibilities for film/video-based therapy. Movie ratings were used to determine which movies were rated the highest around the globe. When the Internet Movie Database was used to collect the top 250 all-time favorite movies, the selections differed with age. Those under 30 have very different assessments from those over 30. While older consumers prefer older movies, younger viewers prefer recent movies. However, consensus did not differ for nationality or culture (Simonton et al., 2012). What we appreciate as viewers is similar across cultures. Based on the research, the implications for cross-cultural video-based therapy are promising; what appeals to one of us appeals to all of us.

References

Agius, T., & Hamer, J. (2003). Thoughts on narrative therapy contribute to Indigenous mental health. *PPEI Magazine, 18*(2), 8–9.

Bandura, A. (Ed.). (1997). *Self-efficacy in changing societies.* Cambridge University Press.

Becker, K. D., Stuewig, J., & McCloskey, L. A. (2010). Traumatic stress symptoms of women exposed to different forms of childhood victimization and intimate partner violence. *Journal of Interpersonal Violence, 25*(9), 1699–1715. doi: 10.1177/0886260509354578

Binder, M. (Writer & Director), Binder, J., Gartner, A., & Lee, S. (Producers). (2005). *The upside of anger* [Film]. Media 8 Entertainment.

Bobkowski, P. S. (2009). Adolescent religiosity and selective exposure to television. *Journal of Media and Religion, 8*(1), 55–70. doi: 10.1080/15348420802670942

Branch, S. E., Wilson, K. M., & Agnew, C. R. (2013, April). Committed to Oprah, Homer or House: Using the investment model to understand parasocial relationships. *Psychology of Popular Media Culture, 2*(2), 96–109. doi: 10.1037/a0030938

Cohen, J. L., Johnson, L. J., & Orr, P. P. (2015). *Video and filmmaking as psychotherapy: Research and practice.* Routledge.

Docter, P. (Director). (2015). *Inside out* [Film]. Pixar Animation Studios.

Erickson, M. H. (1983). *Healing in hypnosis: The seminars, workshops and lectures of Milton H. Erickson* (Vol. 1; Rossi, E. L., Ryan, M. O., & Sharp, F. A. [Eds.]). Irvington.

Heinrich, J., Heine, S. J., & Norenzayan, A. (2010, September). The weirdest people in the world? *Behavioral and Brain Sciences, 33*, 61–83. doi: 10.1017/S0140525X0999152X

Heline, D., & Heiser, E. (Executive Producers). (2009–2018). *The middle* [TV series]. ABC.

IU News Room. (2013). Violent video games may emotionally arouse players. Indiana University Newsletter. https://newsinfo.iu.edu/news-archive/4685.html

Johnson, J. L., & Alderson, K. G. (2008). Therapeutic filmmaking: An exploratory pilot study. *Arts in Psychotherapy, 35*, 11–19. doi: 10.1016/J.AIP.2007.08.004

Krahé, B., Busching, R., & Möller, I. (2012, July). Media violence and aggression among German adolescents: Associations and trajectories of change in a three-wave longitudinal study. *Psychology of Popular Media Culture, 1*(3), 152–166. doi: 10.1037/a0028663

Lippman, J. R., Ward, L. M., & Seabrook, R. C. (2014, July). Isn't it romantic? Differential associations between romantic screen media genres and romantic beliefs. *Psychology of Popular Media Culture, 3*(3), 128–140. doi: 10.1037/ppm0000034

Mramor, N. (1990). *Stress management for children through educational television* (Doctoral dissertation, Saybrook Institute).

Mramor Kajuth, N. (2015). *Get reel: Produce your own life*. Balboa Press.

Neubert, A. P. (2009, October 28). Researchers rest their case: TV consumption predicts behavior about criminal justice system. *Purdue University News Service*. https://www.purdue.edu/newsroom/research/2009/091028SparksCrime.html

Norberg-Hodge, H. (2009). *Ancient futures: Lessons from Ladakh for a globalizing world*. Sierra Club Books.

Simonton, D. K., Graham, J. J., & Kaufman, J. C. (2012, April). Consensus and contrasts in consumers' cinematic assessments: Gender, age, and nationality in rating the top-250 films. *Psychology of Popular Media Culture, 1*(2), 87–96. doi: 10.1037/a0027153

Part IV
Trauma in the World

10 *Chuppah* (*The Wedding Canopy*)
The Holocaust and Trauma

Sascha Schneider

Introduction

They met in the Riga Ghetto in 1942; my mother was deported from Cologne, Germany, and my father was a Latvian, born and raised in Riga. He noticed her when they were all marching out to work, and a few days later slipped her a bar of soap with a note that he would like to meet her. She ran to her parents, who were still alive at the time, and they said, "If he can get the soap to you and the note and still be alive, you should meet him."

So it began. On his birthday, November 7, 1942, he smuggled a bottle of cognac into the German side of the ghetto and proposed to her in front of their parents: "If we stay alive I would like to be with her." They gave their blessing, and my parents considered that their wedding day. They survived the dissolution of the Ghetto, internment in two concentration camps, escape in 1944, and 11 months on the run in the forest. As they often said, "We lost everything and everyone." I was one of the firstborns to the survivors of the Riga Ghetto. We lived with the Holocaust, talked about it, remembered it, and in hindsight tried to deal with the level of trauma and loss by telling the stories.

On my parents' 50th wedding anniversary, we gave them the wedding they never had. As I firmly believe, one cannot deal with the Holocaust without looking at the second and third generations; we therefore put the entire family into the film of that event. For two weeks leading up to the wedding, they told their story of love and survival. The camera captured intimate details of the tensions between brothers, parents and children, wives and in-laws. After the film was shown, won the Santa Barbara Film Festival, and received much praise, I found it fascinating to watch and be part of the healing that occurred in all the family relationships.

We continue to show the film as the centerpiece for healing workshops for children of survivors and other families with historical trauma.

DOI: 10.4324/9781315622507-14

The Upheaval

It was the middle of the night, and the knocking on the door woke every-one up. Helma, the youngest, almost 17, was remembering her lovely dream. They were told to pack only one suitcase per person, leave all valuables behind, and under the watchful eye of the German SS men they were taken out of the apartment. The next thing she could remember was they were herded into a cattle car waiting for the Jews at the station. After two days being squeezed and tossed and lacking all the amenities they grew up with, they arrived in Riga and were escorted to the Ghetto. They were assigned apartments in the "German Ghetto," separated from the "Latvian Ghetto" by barbed wire and a gate guarded by soldiers. There was still food on the table, from the Latvians who were killed to make room for the German Jews.

Every morning the inmates were marched out to work. Benno, by now 19 and the sole survivor of his family (as far as he knew), would line up in the back of the column to make sure he could react "if they started shooting, or something." He was street smart. He had witnessed much of his family being rounded up, and he never saw them again; his father told him to go into hiding while the Germans were "clearing" the Latvian Ghetto.

As they marched, Benno would be aware of his surroundings: the guards, the newcomers from Germany, the women in the column behind his group. Helma Baruch, being a good German girl, lined up alphabetically and marched in the front row. "I liked her," he used to say, so a few days later he slipped her a bar of soap with a note which read, "I would like to meet you." She thought to herself: "If he wants to meet me, he has to meet my parents first." When she got home, she asked her parents what to do, and they said," If he can get soap in the ghetto and not be killed, you should meet him." Thus their courtship began, Benno bribing the guards between the Ghettos and crossing over from one to the other with ease to woo his German girl.

On his birthday, November 7, 1942, Benno came to Helma's house with his uncle and a stolen bottle of cognac, and asked her parents, still alive in the Ghetto, for her hand: "If we survive, I would like to be with her." Her parents blessed the couple and wished them a long life together. They considered it their wedding day, to be remembered and cherished. A couple of months later, Benno, on instinct, told Helma they had to get out of the Ghetto; he could not explain why or what it was that was driving him to go to the ghetto commandant with Helma and ask to be sent to a concentration camp. "Are you crazy?" said the commandant. "We want to go," replied Benno. "OK, go—and see if you survive." Then they were on the way out to the Dundaga concentration camp.

Two weeks later, the Riga Ghetto was eliminated, and almost all the inhabitants murdered, including Helma's parents. The Riga Ghetto was no more.

Dundaga Concentration Camp

Life in camp took an interesting turn; an *oberscharführer*,[1] Wishman, was looking for inmates to work for his section. He was in charge of the supply trains and supplies to the eastern front and was looking for several women to be the cooks and cleaners for the 25 men who loaded and unloaded the trains. As luck would have it, he was from Cologne and heard Helma's Cologne accent. She also credits that the reason he chose her from among the prisoners was that she kept her fingernails clean. From day one, she began to beg Wishman to have Benno join the men in his subcamp. Wishman would respond, "Always 'my Benno'… there are other men here to choose from." After a few weeks Wishman relented, and traded Benno for two bottles of cognac from the camp commander.

Benno became the chauffeur and mechanic for Wishman and his cars. Helma became the fastest potato peeler in the kitchen. As she used to tell us, they were allowed to keep the skin, so she peeled really "heavy" and thick to make sure the soup they made from the potato skins had some heft and flavor.

Benno was in charge of the automobiles, which included the distribution of kerosene from 50-gallon drums. Benno and Wishman would have weekly outings to the farmland around Latvia to make purchases, obtain supplies, etc. During this time, Benno, who spoke fluent Latvian, would make a deal with some of the farmers, trading kerosene for butter, cheese, and eggs, which he brought back to the inmates of the small camp which housed the Wishman Jews. During one of these outings, Benno made contact with an old Latvian farm woman who lived on a small farm alone, as the men were gone into the army or dead.

He made arrangements with the farm woman that she would create a secret shelter for him and Helma that he would keep supplying with provisions, and sometime in the future, they would escape to her, and she would hide them until the war was over. A couple of days before that escape, two of Benno's friends overheard him and Helma, and ran to the older woman's shelter, telling her that Benno had sent them. She took them in, sending word to Benno that they were there, what should she do; she was willing to turn them over to the SS and have Benno and Helma come to stay, but he sent word back, no, I sent them, save them. Both of these men survived, and on one of the significant reunions of the survivors of the Riga Ghetto, as Benno stepped out of a cab at the venue, he met one of these men, who fell on his knees and begged forgiveness; of course, he got it. Benno used to say, "What could I do? We all wanted to live."

One day, Helma spotted the head commandant and a troop of SS guards taking Benno to the wall, where they were going to shoot him. She ran to Wishman, who then ran screaming, "Don't shoot!" He wanted to know why they were about to kill an innocent man. The head commandant responded, "He is a Jew," which meant what does it matter. "He is stealing kerosene." "Let's go see," Wishman insisted, "If anyone is going to shoot him, it will be me. He is my Jew." They opened the kerosene drums to discover that they were full to the top. Benno was spared. He later told Helma that water is denser than kerosene, so he had filled the drums up with water to keep them looking full.

Escape to the Forest

This was life for Benno and Helma until 1944. As the Russian troops were getting closer to the Latvian border, the Germans were liquidating the camps; many prisoners were killed, and the able-bodied were marched to the sea, put onto barges, and transported to Stutthoff for work. On the march, Benno decided with Helma to run, to take a chance in the forest. They passed the message down the line of marching prisoners. When he gave the signal, many ran. Soldiers shot and Benno was hit in the ankle but continued to run into the forest. As Helma was set to run, a young German soldier turned and aimed his rifle at her; she brought up her skirt and squatted down, and as he was raised to be a polite young German, he turned away, and she ran into the forest to meet up with Benno. When they got deeper into the woods, they found five other escapees, including one caught on barbed wire, who Benno freed to join the new family. As luck had it, Mira—on the barbed wire—was a midwife/nurse and healed his wounds and others with herbs they found in the woods. (Later, Helma always used aloe vera for all kinds of scratches, cuts, and burns.) Lotte, one of the five, was pregnant, and Mira delivered a stillborn baby boy a couple of months later. For eleven months, they survived in the woods.

Helma used to say,

> When we were in the woods, we felt free. Never mind we had to be alert to the Germans combing the woods for survivors, the Latvian collaborators, and the Russians; what did I know about them? We were free and in charge of our survival.

Liberation

In the Spring of 1945, Benno woke from a dream in which his mother came to him and said, "Go out, my child, go out." He wandered out into the forest and spotted a Russian patrol. Not sure what to do, Benno made a spur-of-the-moment decision and stood up with his hands raised, speaking Latvian and what Russian he knew. As luck would have it, the lieutenant in charge was Jewish, and they started communicating. They went to get the women, who began running when they saw the uniforms. It took a little time to catch up to them and let them know this was the liberation.

At the relocation camp, Helma was asked if she wanted to go home to Germany. "What about Benno, my husband?" pleaded. She was told, "No, he is Latvian/Soviet and has to stay here." Thus, the decision was made to stay in Riga. They started looking for relatives and friends. They found some friends, miraculously: of the 80,000 Latvian Jews, only 800 survived. They got a bed and their first apartment together, and as Helma said, "no more army boots."

Their first stop was the mayor's office and the official marriage ceremony and certificate. Under the communist system, Jews could not have a religious ceremony, and there was no family and few friends to witness the event. So, there would be no *Chuppah*, no proper Jewish wedding.

Benno got work taking care of trucks and driving for the volunteer fire department in Riga. Helma learned how to cook and how to speak Russian and Latvian, and she had to learn Yiddish as that was the language of choice by the survivors when they got together.

The Next Generation

I was born in May of 1946, one of the firstborn children to the survivors of the Riga Ghetto. This has been my moniker for most of my life; as my parents so often told me, I was their blessing and the ultimate revenge on Hitler. My father often reflected on why he survived while the rest of his family members were killed, and he decided that the reason he was alive was to tell the stories and to bear witness. From a very early age, I was the recipient of my father's detailed stories of his and my mother's experiences during the Holocaust. The stories became mine, for whom better to tell all than the firstborn male? Life started to normalize, Benno began playing tennis again, and became the Latvian champion. He was beginning to make money in the Soviet system of "working to the left": i.e., one for the government and one for me.

As a child, I was aware that my parents were "different." There were moments in which both Benno and Helma had no way of coping. What I saw were tears, anger, frustration, and ultimately the two of them in an embrace, letting the "thing" go by. The trauma was palpable.

Benno's Arrest

Then came a night in 1952. The KGB came to the door at 3:00 a.m. and took Benno away while the house was searched and some money taken. By the time Helma got to the police station, it was too late: Benno was gone. In the past, she was always able to "buy" him out, but this time he was already on a train to the Gulag. We had no idea where, for how long, and what, if any, the charges were. Our assumption was that he was involved with the black market, in which the majority of the population participated.

During these two years, I became the "man" of the house—I was Mom's confidant, caretaker, and support. As I usually point out, "I was never a child": Mom needed someone to talk to, share with, and bring up the wood for the stove, take care of the dog, shop, and help her cook.

My orders were never to divulge what was said or done in the house, be a presence in the outside world, be a good young pioneer and follow the track toward the communist party, and always remember you are a Jew, a child of survivors, but don't confuse the two, and be clear whom you can trust, only blood.

My father came back two years later, a bit thinner and a bit darker. Still, he guided us all to a reasonably healthy life. He loved to laugh, have friends over, and, whenever possible, to help others.

A Reunion

I learned the lesson from my parents to "Always be careful, but risk reaching for life, for the risk is always worth it." Many of the stories of my childhood had to do with my dad's risk-taking to save himself, Mom, and many others in the ghetto, camp, and the forest. One particular story comes to mind. In New York, my wife, my parents, and I attended the 45th reunion of the survivors of the Riga Ghetto. It was beautiful to see the survivors greeting each other as if they were still young, flirtatious, and whole. They had survived. A man about eight years older than I came over to me, looked at my name tag, and said,

> I was a child from Kassel, and when we got to Riga, the children without parents were all put into a barbed-wire enclosure in the hope that we would all starve to death. Some were beginning to die. And then one day, a truck pulled up and a man in a German uniform got out and began throwing sandwiches and water over the barbed wire. Many of us got stronger, and the Germans decided to put us to work, and that is how I survived. Later we found out that it wasn't a German soldier but one of us, an inmate, a Jew who drove the truck and wore the uniform. Somehow he had gotten all that food and water for us. His name was Benno Schneider. We heard that he was killed.

I told the man, "Benno Schneider is my father, and not only is he alive, but he is also right there in the room." You can only imagine the reunion between this young man and my father.

Relocation

In 1958, Germany and the Soviet Union made an agreement that those who could prove that they had been German citizens until 1941 could take their family and go home to Germany. We had long discussions: "Is this real? Are the Soviets to be trusted?" And finally, a good friend of my father, who was the chief of the traffic police in Riga, told him that "his number might be up again." He couldn't survive the Gulag again, so the decision was clear. Mom went to Moscow, filed the official papers, put some money on the table (and some under), and presented her Cologne, Germany, birth certificate, which had been sent to us by her cousins, who were back living in Germany.

Much later, we got our permission to immigrate and then came the long goodbyes, the packing, the decisions of what to take and how—legal or otherwise. We were allowed some cash for each family member, but certainly not all the cash Dad had, so he bought gold coins, some mink pelts, and anything else he thought would be "money" in Germany.

We were now four: my mother, father, and three-year-old brother and myself. We arrived in the large railroad station hall in Brest Litovsk, on the Polish border. I still have a vivid memory of the empty hall, putting our luggage atop a long table for the border guards to open and thoroughly examine. There was one exit with one train car, no markings visible, and four border patrol guards with dogs and machine guns at the exit. They took all our documents away, marked the suitcases, walked us past the dogs and guards into the train compartment, and closed the door. Mom's first reaction was, "Where are we going? It could be Siberia, or somewhere else." As the train began to move, an officer came in, returned our passports and travel documents, and left the compartment. It was not until we got to the Polish border and the exchange of locomotives that we felt a bit safer, as we were now moving through Poland into Germany.

Next stop, Berlin. What a fantastic shock to come from the Soviet Union to West Germany. We settled in Frankfurt am/Main. We thought that was the final stop. Alas, it was not to be. As Mom was registering me into a "Humanistishes Gymnasium," we were sitting with the school principal, and he told her, "Since Sascha is not going to have religion class, when the children ask what religion he is, have him say none." "And why would he do that?" she asked. "Well," came the reply, "you never know what is still in the hearts of the German people." When we got home, she was very clear that even though Germany was her birthplace, she could not live here. Every time she saw a man ten or so years older, she would ask herself, "What did you do? Did you kill my family?"

It was 1961 when we finally got our visas to the U.S., the real Promised Land, and in April we were on our way to Los Angeles.

Immigration

The U.S. was my father's world. He could do all things he did in the Soviet Union, but here he would not be arrested for going downtown on Saturdays to buy socks, t-shirts, or shoes, and sell them to his coworkers for a bit of a profit. We saved and saved, and he purchased his first business, a delicatessen. It was a family business where we all had to pitch in and work,

Our family *shtetl* was being created. Finally, in 1975, my dad built a five-unit apartment house, and he and Mom moved into the front apartment, which had been created for them. Years later, my brother and his wife moved into the back unit with their son and daughter. Nothing made my mother happier than to have everyone so close and safe. My brother was delighted too because his children had grandparents close by, which he had never known.

Mom was in control, and all life around the building, including the tenants, went through her. If she did not have control, her anxiety grew, and we all felt it.

For most of my life, the messages were obvious

You have to save 6 million. We are the revenge on Hitler, the future of Jews in the world. Make sure your parents are safe and happy, and never angry or disappointed. Keep the family first, don't trust anyone but family, and, most of all, don't abandon the family.

When I moved out, my brother and his wife felt they could not hurt my parents and thus stayed in the building, "within spitting distance" of Mom and Dad's influence. Through all the years in Los Angeles, Mom and Dad continued to impress on us the fact that in 40 years they had never had a real wedding. The persistent message was that it would be amazing to have a *Chuppah*: "Would the dead relatives not be happy and at peace? Wouldn't it be a real gift to our survival?"

Now there was family: my brother, his wife, and two children; me, my wife, and one child; so, the *Chuppah* would be witnessed and blessed. In 1992, we decided to give them a *Chuppah* and planned to do the ceremony on November 7, Dad's birthday, 50 years from the night Dad asked Mom's parents for her hand, and the day they considered to be their wedding anniversary.

Making the Film

"We make plans, and God laughs."[2] As the world would have it, that same year, I got a job in Germany and moved my family to Berlin. We continued the preparations for the *Chuppah*. Since my wife and I were both filmmakers, we decided to make a documentary about my parents' story and the wedding. As luck would have it, while in Berlin, we met the head of the documentary division for UFA films, and he got very interested in the story. My wife wrote a proposal, and the division committed to fund half the money to do the movie. My wife returned to Los Angeles, weeks ahead of the date, and we were able to hire a beautiful, caring, and talented cinematographer, Hanania Baer, for the filming, as well as a great sound man. Eight days before the wedding, we began the telling of the story.

I do not believe one can tell the story of survivors without including the second generation and beyond, as transgenerational trauma has been documented to travel for several generations (Danieli, 1998, 2007). We intended to make sure that everyone in the family got their chance to tell their story of growing up in this highly traumatized family, the way they felt, growing up, now, and what this *Chuppah* meant to them. We also began Mom and Dad's story from the beginning: Mom growing up as the youngest of a large tribe of Baruchs in Cologne, Germany; Dad from his youth in Riga, his yeshiva studies, and his father's insistence that he learn something practical, becoming an auto mechanic. Everyone got used to the camera and opened up to their feelings. We filmed at every opportunity to get to the depth of the story and the family experiences and perceptions of life together. Family drama unfolded around the event of the wedding. My wife was pregnant with a boy, and she and I debated whether to do a *bris*[3] and whether my parents would return to Germany for our son's birth. The family conflicts ran deep against the grain of their story: How could we deny a tradition that many had died for; how could we set boundaries where family bonds are everything; and how could my brother and his family contemplate moving away when his parents had lost their whole family? We finished filming the day of the *Chuppah* ceremony, with these many questions remaining,

We went back to Germany, hired an excellent German editor, and began work on the film. While in Berlin, we decided to go through with the circumcision and contacted the local *mohel*[4] to do the ceremony. Unfortunately, a month before the birth of my son, he got hepatitis B and quit that profession. Our only remaining choice was the Jewish Hospital in Berlin, as a surgical procedure. Mom and Dad came to Berlin, and while it was not the most spiritual of settings, Dad got to sing the prayers while holding my son, as our friends, dressed entirely in surgical blues, looked on from one side of the surgical suite and about 17 interns dressed in surgical greens observed from the other side. They had never witnessed a circumcision.

The story of the film culminates in Germany with our son's birth and my parents' visit.

Screening the Film

We returned to Los Angeles to finish the film: we mixed it, color-timed it, and finally had a DVD to show. It took a few weeks to drum up our courage to show it to the family, as it was not all roses and joy. We asked friends and the cinematographer to come to the screening as buffers. The film ran for 80 minutes and then there was silence. My sister-in-law was the first to ask, "How come you used these stories and left others out?" My dad chimed in, "Well, what about this story, and that story, and did you have to show all of us in disagreement and pain?"

We submitted the documentary to several film festivals. The Santa Barbara Film Festival was our first acceptance. They scheduled two screenings, both of which were packed to the brim, standing room only. After the first screening, there was a Q&A, and I asked Mom and Dad to come up. As they walked to the stage, there was a long, standing ovation; people were crying and cheering. My father turned to me and said, "You changed the film. Well done." Of course, we did not touch a frame, but the relief on his face was evident: the story was finally out and immortalized. He had succeeded in his life mission, and his oldest son had done his duty to continue the legacy.

A Healing Effect

This public airing of my parents' story and family conflicts had a healing effect on all our relationships. Shortly after the screening in Santa Barbara, my brother took the giant step to move into his own house with his family, and this time our parents were supportive and helpful. My mother came to my wife and me and asked us to take her to a psychotherapist: she felt depressed, dark, and not herself. We found a Hungarian psychiatrist who was a survivor himself, perfectly cast as he looked over the spectacles on his nose and spoke to my mother in a thick European accent. She felt understood and accepted his prescription of a mild antidepressant. They had three sessions, and she became a different person, more joyous and positive. We had not experienced her with so much laughter. When the pills ran out, she informed us that the psychiatrist was too expensive, and the pills did nothing for her, and she went back under the dark cloud. She could not let go of suffering, as it would "betray" her dead family. Yet the fact that the story was publicly told seemed to lighten the load. Mom was able to look at the demons that had been holding her back from loving relationships with her daughters-in-law, and we all found common ground, more joy together as well as healthier separation.

The film was a labor of love that created healing in our family beyond our expectations. My wife and I began to present workshops for survivors as well as the second and third generations of individuals and couples. We followed screenings of the film with a workshop. The film triggered various feelings about internal struggles and difficulties in relationships that people then shared. Using the film as a centerpiece, we were able to help other families and individuals to confront and heal many Holocaust-related issues and trauma.

Notes

1 A Nazi senior squad leader.
2 Old Yiddish proverb.

3 The Jewish ritual of circumcision.
4 A doctor or rabbi trained in the rituals and practice of performing circumcisions.

References

Danieli, Y. (Ed.). (1998). *International handbook of multigenerational legacies of trauma*. Plenum Press.

Danieli, Y. (2007). Assessing trauma across cultures from a multigenerational perspective. In J. P. Wilson & C. S.-K. Tang (Eds.), *Cross-cultural assessment of psychological trauma and PTSD* (pp. 65–89). Springer Science + Business Media. doi: 10.1007/978-0-387-70990-1_4

11 Video Movie Therapy (VMT) Psychotherapy

Gaetano Giordano

Introduction

With the term Video Movie Therapy (VMT), we refer to a planned system of intervention for the treatment of mental illness. This system, implemented within a therapeutic relationship, can be applied to reduce symptoms of psychological distress or to modify basic personality structure.

VMT is a type of group psychotherapy aimed at treating psychological disorders and some psychiatric pathologies and draws from the creative and self-referential potentialities of video recordings. It began to develop in April 1987 and, according to Judy Weiser (2019), is a uniquely creative use of videos and movies made by clients during their treatment.

The aim of the group is the production (from screenplay to post-editing) of a movie or of a short series of 60-minute episodes, in which each group participant (therapist included) will play his or her own "character"; the character will have the same name, profession, sociocultural background, and marital status as the patient who plays the part. The plot will be based on an ironic take on the group, on therapy, and on the specific stories of the single participants, in an attempt to produce an experience in which the difference between set and setting, actor and character cancel that which is denied at one level is expressed at another. This activity enables participants to become aware of how each one actively constructs his or her reality (McLeod, 2019).

In Italy, every movie should be inspired by the classic "Italian comedy," or better yet, the classic movies from the 1960s with leading comical actors such as Alberto Sordi and Totò.

VMT Technique and Setting

The VMT group, usually made up of five to seven patients, aims at producing a 90-minute movie, or a mini-series of two to four 60-minute episodes, about a story whose characters are those of the actors who impersonate them. For example, if Dr. Giordano is the group's

DOI: 10.4324/9781315622507-15

psychotherapist, and Mr. Smith and Mrs. Jane are two group participants, Dr. Giordano will play the role of "Dr. Giordano," psychotherapist, who is currently treating the characters of the film. The characters will have the same profession and the same family and relationship status as that of the participants who impersonate them. The story is set in the therapist's office and, when possible, in the participants' homes, provided this does not violate the intimacy and confidentiality of the patients or of their family members (who, in some cases, may participate in the production).

This author strictly recommends that all VMT group participants already be following an analytic therapy, either with the group conductor or with another referred psychotherapist. In some cases, the VMT group therapist and the individual therapist should be different.

The "movie" created by the group should have an ironic or comical style (even if some dramatic moments will be unavoidable), and the general tone of all participants should be that of benevolent irony.

The group meetings start with an individual meeting in which each participant is informed about the practice, the rules, the philosophy of VMT, the character he or she will play, and the limits of this interpretation.

There is no preassigned script or subject: the group will periodically decide the story and script development. Any group participant can propose whichever aspect of the film they choose, ranging from story development to individual scenes to dialogues, director's notes, costumes, setting, and more. Every decision is made through group discussion. It is essential that the psychotherapist refrain from psychoanalytic interpretations, even if close attention is on the ongoing individual and group dynamics. Participants in a VMT group are extremely sensitive to feeling exposed, due to their lack of self-esteem or their guilt feelings; in this context, the therapist displays a benevolent and caring attitude, carefully avoiding sarcasm or "excessive" irony.

It is mandatory that any form of physical contact, be it affectionate or violent, between the "actors/patients" be avoided. No scenes involving physical contact are permitted, neither kissing nor any behavior which, in the given sociocultural context, marks the beginning of a possible physical (again, be it violent or affectionate) interaction.

The therapist encourages the group to promote and define all aspects of the subject development from the construction of the individual scenes, to acting, writing the director's notes, and so forth, as described above. The therapist's interventions should stimulate the participants to best express their character through acting, and the therapist may make suggestions to further the subjects' development, always making sure that this is done primarily by the participants themselves. The therapist manages and elaborates on any destructive and/or aggressive process that may arise within the group; for example, it is likely that aggression and "shadow attacks" may express themselves through the participants' suggestions and comments relating to the creation of the subject and its staging. Anything of this kind that arises during the sessions is processed in the individual sessions with each patient. From this point of view, it is best to consider VMT as joint therapy (if group therapist and individual therapist are different) or as "multiple-setting" therapy (if group conductor and individual therapist are the same person).

In summary, irony and creativity can be very useful and efficient tools in the management of psychological distress, but they should be used with caution by the group therapist.

VMT setting rules are critical because they are what makes the VMT experience therapeutic. Given that the group performance centers on all that is ironic and funny, it is important that self-reflection defines the context within which group members interact. It is also important to define a clear sense of commitment for the context within which participants interact.

Additionally, the VMT setting requires weekly meetings; depending on the scene requirements, meetings may last from 90 minutes to 2 hours. Absent patients are still required to pay for a missed session. Nothing of what is said and done within the group is allowed in discussions outside of the group itself. The therapist does not make any copies of the movie, and its viewing is reserved exclusively to the assembled group as such. Editing and post-production are done within group sessions; after editing, three or four group sessions are devoted to viewing and commenting on the final video. During these commentary sessions, problems of the individual participants will be addressed. There is no required maximum number of sessions to complete the film.

The result of a VMT group should be—in cinematography terms—as close as possible to a "good movie," yet this should not occur at the expense of the participants, who should all be able to express themselves adequately. Note that, in implementing VMT practice, it will always be necessary to balance the desire to "make a good movie" with the necessity of allowing space for the expressive and psychotherapeutic needs of each participant. Another point of VMT is to allow room to work on the therapeutic aspects. These aspects can emerge simply from working on the development of the movie itself. All participants should be informed and reminded of this, especially when making decisions regarding the development of the subject or the screenplay, to avoid repetition and lengthy scenes or narratives.

The effort to approximate a functional "cinematography language" is, in fact, a crucial aspect of VMT, and it contributes significantly in defining both its therapeutic potential and its capacity. The act of "representing themselves" should not merely mirror everyday behaviors; rather, it should be the result of a reflection—a study—of one's way of being and behaving. It should be a "distillation" of elaborating behaviors during therapy sessions: the most characteristic traits become those same traits which give life to a character.

From this perspective, it is essential to distance oneself from the expectation of being a great producer and creating a beautiful movie. Instead, it is crucial to achieve a useful cinematography language, as this activates one of the therapeutic aspects of VMT and is framed in this light.

The definition of a movie "character," and their interactions with the other characters, is brought about through an intensive effort at contextualization and definition of the participants' assumptions, of the way they think, judge, and act, the way they legitimize themselves toward their selves and the world. Subsequently, all this is "re-written" in a synopsis of behaviors and interactive modes that highlight the characters' manners, values, and perspectives. This process requires that the actor/participant be able to "distill" their life flow into a series of characteristics, connotations, and features, and to reduce and process them (with the help of the other participants) in an expressive synthesis with metaphorical capacities.

The creation of the various narrative links and individual scenes will enable participants to perceive how their narration reflects what each "character" builds and defines as their own "reality," and how the "self" uses "objectivity" to legitimize and confirm its functioning and its understanding of "objectivity." We are referring here to the work of Maturana and Varela (1980, 1998); the working hypothesis is that the construction of the set/setting will implicitly lead those who take part in it to experience that the difference between "perception" and "illusion" is a post hoc explanation given by the observer. Furthermore, participants will experience that their so-called reality, the Self, and self-awareness exist in language as an explanation of the immediate experience of the observer, and these concepts always assume the premises in which they are "objectified" by the observer.

To express, in a three-minute video scene, the salient characteristics of one's way of being, it is necessary to study and summarize one's assumptions to provide the actor with a "map" of himself or herself, a map which is necessary to express one's own character in a significant metaphorical and summarized way. For example, hypochondriac, anxious, or obsessive traits must be initially contextualized as such, then rewritten in such a way that they express, through the synthesized movie metaphor, the self-referentiality.

Whereas in daily life the ego legitimizes the reasons for its functioning through "objectivity," in the movie construction experienced in VMT the reverse is true: given a series of characteristics and perspectives, the participants create events and narrative moments which express how each individual legitimizes their way of responding to events. Individual responses will be consistent with a participant's premises and assumptions and will legitimize their way of perceiving "reality" as "reality" and not, in fact, as a construction.

In summary, the search for an appropriate film language enables participants to perceive in which measure the "ego" uses "objectivity" to continue to operate, legitimizing its premises and perspectives. The synthesis—necessary to condense the character's personality into a scene and in film language—implies that the ego (or the Self, depending on our reader's viewpoint) is the starting point of the relationship between the "ego" (or the self) of the "character" and what they call "reality" rather than "objectivity."

Essentially this is the "core" experience which, in VMT practice, enables group participants to become aware that everyone is mostly the character he or she decides to be, constructing events that confirm this same perception.

It is clear, from this point of view, that being able to create a "good movie"—which, moreover, nobody will see—becomes a zen-like task (think of a Japanese zen garden) because it requires a balance between irony, self-reflection, and creative skills which are necessary to participate.

Epistemological and Psychotherapeutic Grounds of VMT

VMT encompasses several different epistemological and psychotherapeutic premises. Classic Greek and Roman theater aimed at the "catharsis" of public passions, what Aristotle defined as "purging of the spirit of morbid and basic ideas or emotions by witnessing the playing out of such emotions or ideas on stage" (Powell, n.d., para. 1). The concept of catharsis is not new to psychology and psychotherapy; it can be traced to the dawning of psychoanalysis, and the therapeutic moment in psychoanalysis closely resembles catharsis.

From this standpoint, we can't ignore that many so-called models of "strategic therapies" are also based—directly or indirectly—on the repetition or revisiting via a script (and therefore, if you will, the "staging") of the presenting symptom (for example, so-called "symptom prescription"). In summary, it appears that in most psychotherapies distress will endure until the Ego becomes aware of the difference between the "map" and the "territory" (to use a familiar image).

Another concept which VMT refers to is what Bateson (1999) defined as "transcontextual" experiences such as games, theater, psychotherapy, and irony, and in this quality resides the therapeutic value of psychotherapy. Another crucial theoretical premise of VMT is found in the studies of Maturana and Varela (1980, 1998), who—according to Bateson himself—carried on Bateson's work further. An additional and important assumption of VMT is that the healing power of therapy resides not so much in techniques or strategies, but preferably in the ethics with which they are implemented.

"Ethics" refers to the psychotherapist's ability to apply the technique and the practice they deem is most consistent with their operational concept of "therapist." These must necessarily include respect for the patient's illness, sharing of the patient's grief, and the patient's willingness to heal according to therapy goals. Goals are based not on the therapist's concept of health but on what is consistent with the patient's requests, expectations, personality, and status.

Conditions, Pathologies, and Contexts of Distress in Which VMT May Be Used

VMT can be used only in cases that fall within a specific clinical and psychological profile, responding to the following criteria:

- Unsolicited request for psychotherapy
- Diagnosis of neurotic disorder or personality; absence of psychosis or so-called psychotic disorders; full competency of the patient
- The "patient" displays a tendency to express problems by "acting out" behaviors but retains the capacity to reflect on the meaning of the same; displays a reasonable degree of extroversion and communication skills; is capable of self-irony

In our experience and statistics, following pathologies respond very well to this practice:

- Anxiety disorders, including panic disorder; obsessive-phobic forms
- Depressive syndromes of psychogenic origin
- Post-traumatic stress disorders (PTSDs)

Personality disorders seem to respond differently depending on the patient, so particular caution must be used, especially for pathologies that once would have fallen under the label of passive-aggressive personality disorder.

Among post-traumatic stress disorders, we also currently include—saving later revisions—so-called parental alienation problems, which may be diagnosed as cases of so-called Parental Alienation Syndrome (PAS). See below for a more in-depth discussion of PAS.

Application of VMT to Post-Traumatic Stress Syndrome

PTSD presents an exception to the typical context of the application of VMT. The patients we have followed with this syndrome include war or conflict survivors, women victims of domestic violence, victims of car accidents, and patients mourning the death of a loved one through a car accident. In these cases, VMT methodology must be radically changed. It is barely appropriate to request self-irony from a patient suffering from PTSD: one might perceive this as a lack of respect and understanding. It is, however, clear that a person recovering from a traumatic experience can improve if and when they can be ironic about the situation.

In this sense, the role of the psychotherapist can be vital in understanding that irony is not a way to ridicule patients and their discomfort;

rather, it is an affectionate attempt to share a problem and its solution. We are referring here to the world of Zen, in which a monk laughs when he realizes that everything (including this statement) is an illusion. In this light, psychotherapists are always "frauds" who look after their patients by attempting to deceive them; the basic idea is that "theories" always present a risk of deception if their use is not supported by a behavior that is both ethical and, to use a Buddhist term, "compassionate."

Regarding post-traumatic syndromes, although lacking the element of irony, the main rule remains unchanged: the real story must be presented in a narrative context which gives it a different connotation. PTSD subjects will therefore—depending on the other participants—be able to impersonate either the role of a psychotherapist who is treating a subject suffering from PTSD (in turn interpreted by the therapist who leads the groups), or that of a writer, director, or actor who must work with PTSD-related stories. In this sense, the stories of the other participants can be ironically redescribed as traumatizing, even if the element of trauma is entirely absent from the reality and can be made to interact with the stories of the PTSD participant. For example, this approach is being used with a young man who had fallen behind in his studies due to his "depression." In the video recording, his "going to classes every day" and "taking exams" were redescribed as a severe trauma experienced by the character. Another patient affected by chronic PTSD (connected to his military experiences in war zones) was assigned the role of a psychologist who had to help the student without causing him "too much suffering." To do this, the student had to "train" by enacting some scenes—under the veteran's instructions—in which the latter had been a protagonist during the war. We observed that the student's narcissism, like his inability to complete projects, suffered a big shock.

It is essential, at this point, to shed light on an important aspect: the construction of VMT events can make use of moralistic interpretative stereotypes. The interpretation given to these by the group psychotherapist would be different, but the use of these stereotypes is designed to make the participants confront their guilt feelings.

Application of VMT to "Parental Alienation Syndrome"

Parental alienation syndromes, the nosographic dignity of which, in Italy, is still an object of discussion, deserve an entirely separate intervention. Regarding VMT, the conflictual parent context is considered a highly traumatic environment for the child, and the refusal on behalf of the child to meet one of their parents is considered a particular form of PTSD. It must be noted that this classification is not in the *DSM* or, at this time, in any other literature.

To this day, only parents are allowed to participate in VMT groups as the experience is excessively traumatic for children. Both the experience of the parent who is rejected by the child ("the alienated parent") and the situation which leads the child to reject one parent are considered traumatic experiences. "Alienated parents" (with all due care for individual sensibility) are asked to act the part of a parent (and represent a caricature of one) who behaves precisely as the children accuse him or her of really behaving (in the group, this parent can be assigned a child, played by another participant who has conflicts with his/her parents). This conflict often helps the participants diminish the sense of internal persecution and can miraculously defuse it. The other aspect which we attempt to change is the parents' empathic capacity toward their children, which "alienated" parents are often missing, constantly or temporarily because of the ongoing conflict.

A golden rule of VMT is always to encourage alienated parents to consider their children's expectations as a priority. Another effort usually made in this context is that of giving the story a historical perspective; most separated parents with serious conflictual separation problems cannot imagine how the situation will evolve. They are anchored to a pathological here and now, and quickly forget that in a few years (and in this sense, the length of court proceedings has an even more adverse effect on the situation) the children's age and changing situations will create a different context. The crux is therefore to think about what the relationship with those children will be like in the future, rather than in the here and now. To emphasize this fundamental aspect, we try to structure a narrative hypothesis that may describe these kinds of developments.

Other Applications of VMT

Interventions in Marital Conflict

Following the logic of VMT, in cases of marital discord there is a paradoxical enactment of the conflict: the "Court" is transposed to the psychotherapist's study and, using the "conflict" to manage the conflict, the psychotherapist becomes "the judge," and other patients represent the spouses' "attorneys." The couple will have to present their situation, bringing evidence and "memoirs," again with the help of their attorneys. Each "memoir" is about 30 pages long and can be assigned as a task by the therapist.

The sessions (excluding children) in these cases can last up to two hours (even two and a half, if the therapist is available), and are likely strenuous. It must be explained beforehand ("Conflict comes at a price") that the therapist's meter will continue running for the duration of the session ("The more you quarrel, the more others will profit from it!").

Every session is centered on the ironic dramatization of the persecutory ghosts of the partners: the therapist works hard to find new faults with the spouses and will produce exasperating harangues against both, demanding new evidence and proof. Every so often the therapist—as judge—will pronounce a decree containing a paradoxical prescription.

Several paradoxical strategies are possible: the "Charges contest," for example, during which both partners must, in turn, fill the other with accusations, without reference to facts but to allegedly "objective" data. The player who manages to talk for the longest time or who remains unmoved by the accusations wins. Usually, after a few similar "contests," spouses become aware of how they are just repeating the same few concepts, and of how they do not know how to fight without each other's help.

Some other paradoxical prescriptions may be "assigned arguing" (for a fixed duration, even at night, at preestablished times), a "grievances contest", "resistance tests" based on applying the children's visitation rights granted to one spouse to the other spouse, and so forth. The aim is to succeed in ensuring that the real strategies, which the couple reverts to during the conflict, become exasperating and paradoxical; thus, it will become impossible for the spouses to quarrel about formalizing agreements which were already implicitly made.

Motion Capture

One of our colleagues, V. De Laurentiis, is considering a possible setting for children, rooted in VMT's working hypothesis, based on "Motion Capture" technology. This approach would undoubtedly open new frontiers, and, although the application of this technology does not appear to be immediately or easily accessible, when it is implemented it will likely meet with much praise.

Other Creative Environments

VMT's operating code (if we want to call it that) can be applied to various creative contexts which we have attempted to use from time to time; among these we record the "Photo Story" and theater script writing.

Conclusion

To conclude, we would like to summarize in a few lines what we are saying thus far. VMT is a system based on the "therapeutic" effectiveness of "acting a scene": in other words, of expressing, in a transcontextual dimension, human distress and the problems resulting from it, and the possibility offered by irony which allows one to discover solutions where previously one could only see problems. An iron rule which, according to this author, should warrant the therapeutic efficacy of this treatment and all other psychotherapies is that it is applied according to strict ethical standards.

References

Bateson, G. (1999). *Steps to an ecology of mind: Collected essays in anthropology, psychiatry, evolution, and epistemology*. Jason Aronson. doi: 10.7208/chicago/9780226924601.001.0001

Maturana, H. R., & Varela, F. J. (1980). *Autopoiesis and cognition: The realization of the living*. Reidel Publishing.

Maturana, H. R., & Varela, F. J. (1998). *The tree of knowledge: The biological roots of human understanding* (Rev. ed.). Shambhala.

McLeod, S. A. (2019, July 17). Constructivism *as a theory for teaching and learning*. Simply Psychology. www.simplypsychology.org/constructivism.html

Powell, E. (n.d.). Catharsis in psychology and beyond: A historic overview. *The Primal Psychotherapy Page Index*. http://primal-page.com/cathar.htm

Weiser, J. (2019). *Phototherapy techniques: Exploring the secrets of personal snapshots and family albums*. Routledge.

12 Directing with the "Gaze"[1]

Video Art Therapy as Viewed from Gestalt Therapy, Psychoanalysis, and Holism

Rodríguez Pérez, R. N.

An Introduction to Video as a Creative Tool in Art Therapy

Like other new technologies, video brings a new materiality to works of art and a new means of developing insights into how they are produced. The multiple dimensions of time, space, and sound, along with the ability to pause, visit, or view an artwork or view it in conjunction with others and allow video to operate on a different level to sculpture, painting, or photography, while nevertheless being informed by these fields. These characteristics enable the medium to generate a new language, different but equally valid to those of the aforementioned traditions.

Video does not merely provide us with an image of reality. It gives us a view, which is conditioned by the person who films, edits, and observes that reality, and, of course, by the subject of the production.[2] This is what makes video's use in art therapy of such interest: the medium allows people to work with their self-image or with their way of seeing the world; later it gives them the chance to view what they have filmed or even to show it to others.

The four fundamental elements in the process of video art therapy sessions are filming, viewing, editing, and analysis of that which has been produced. The "gaze" of those who film is present at each of these stages: it is involved in the process of decision-making, direction, and choosing between alternative paths. It is therefore important to understand what happens in the process of looking, viewing, and interpreting by following the path of the participants' gaze. The use of the concept "gaze" in this chapter refers to its treatment in the fields of psychoanalysis, Gestalt psychotherapy, and holism.

An example of the creative and therapeutic process that patients experience in the sessions is the moment at which a patient takes hold of the camera. At this point, using the input from the therapist as a springboard (such as a phrase, an image, or a song), the patient positions the camera, decides what to focus on, and starts to film. Nothing is filmed by chance: the patient chooses one part of reality, and the rest is thereby excluded. They frame a shot, focus the camera on something, move closer

DOI: 10.4324/9781315622507-16

or draw away from it, vary the speed, and pause. Later on, they view what they have filmed and imagine a story, characters, and perhaps music. Then it's time to edit, think symbolically, and play with the images by cutting them, speeding them up or slowing them down, changing them to black and white, repeating scenes, combining screens, distorting shots, changing the tone, making transitions, and adding sound, music, subtitles, fixed images, or maps.

Video art therapy process allows the patient to start expanding their perspective, their position in the world, and their view of the current reality. Video art tools are very powerful, and it is worth adapting their use to art therapy practice. Video is, for example, an incredible tool to use with children and teenagers because the video camera allows them to show their vision (working with their self-image). It gives a role and a presence to the person while recording, granting a space to their gaze and letting them make decisions. It also provides a position for those who are recorded. Its use also implies the importance of knowing and respecting certain rules: basic operation of the camera, and respect for another person's image and for what they want to show and what they do not.

The Place of Video in art Therapy Sessions

> I do not intend to affirm that I have always been respectful of the truth of my narration. I have exaggerated, added, removed and changed the order, but, as usually happens in this type of games, the game has turned out to be surely clearer than reality.
>
> (Bergman, 1992, p. 10)

Fundamental in attempting to define art therapy and exploring video's role in this field was gaining an understanding of how different professionals engage in practice, identifying the unique possibilities that this tool offers, and exploring how sessions were framed. Through this process, it has been possible to construct a broad overview of the history of video art therapy.

Conducting a survey of the number of professionals working in video therapy and video art therapy gave a clearer picture of the current state of the field. This stage of my research provided evidence that video is a growing area in clinical use, as well as in the fields of art therapy and psychotherapy. Most of the researchers and professionals who work in this field live in the United States, England, Canada, Switzerland, Spain, France, and Italy.

With regard to the situation in Spain, the incorporation of video into art therapy practice has become increasingly common, particularly in the last decade, although it has still had little impact on the content of art therapy courses in Spanish universities. An exception is the video art therapy module delivered by Dr. Ana Mampaso since 2001 as part of the interuniversity master's program in Art Therapy and Artistic Education for Social Inclusion (the Complutense University of Madrid and the Autonomous University of Madrid) (Mampaso Martínez, 2001, 2004). Different private courses have also been developed, such as the "Video Therapy, Cinema Therapy, and Video Art Therapy" program coordinated by Olga Rueda in Madrid (Rueda Cuenca, 2010, 2018). Elsewhere in Europe, the most significant program found was the master's in "Video, Photography, Theatre and Artistic Mediation in Care Relationships" offered by the Pontifical University Antonianum in Rome.

In countries where art therapy is not a law-regulated activity, such as Spain, creating a solid framework for the video art therapy field initially seems a challenging task, given its emphasis on viewing the person holistically rather than treating specific symptoms. A clear definition of video art therapy is vital if the field's potential is to be realized, as will identifying the specific contributions that it can make and establishing exactly how the process of professional accreditation will work, including recognizing an accrediting body.

As a first step in building this framework, video art therapy may be defined as a therapeutic intervention which employs audiovisual language as a creative tool for patients' use in the sessions. The patient's development is observed through the change in their "gaze": the way in which they view and direct the production process. By transforming the production through screening, editing, and analysis, patients develop an increasing number of ways of viewing their film. Through this process, the range of ways in which they see the world and themselves will also increase.

When choosing from different methodological options for art therapy practice, the aim is not to identify one method to fit all cases. Nor is it to create an empirically measurable model to which video art therapists must adapt their work, particularly in contexts in which practice is not yet regulated. Instead, the emphasis must be on providing art therapy practice with credibility, which makes it crucial to establish a process for identifying and certifying professionals. This process should account for such factors as: training, the number of hours of supervised and unsupervised practice (including personal therapy practice), research, publications, and conference presentations. So, we can avoid a definition of "intervention in the field" that is too narrow.

Art, including that realized in video, has been shown to have enormous potential in therapy for exploring the realms of the unconscious and desire, helping to uncover that which is hidden or denied, and breaking down patients' barriers. Spoken discourse, which usually passes through the filter of cognitive processes, is somehow more diffuse, clouded, and confused. Art is a direct manifestation of the symbolic universe, of the worlds of our desires, dreams, imagination, and memories; and these can be expressed more directly through the body, the emotions, and the spiritual self.

To reach a fuller understanding of video as a creative tool in art therapy sessions, it is important to acknowledge the equally valuable role played by each stage of videography (filming, viewing, editing, and analysis) in the production process.

The externalization of patients' subjective view of the world (in that which is captured on film) enables patients to consider this vision from a distance and gives video art therapists clues as to how to develop their intervention. With access to products of the patient's imagination, the therapist can proceed with reference to their choices of shot, light, color, etc.

Perception is defined as a sensory phenomenon, an act which is unique to each one of us, while the "gaze" is characterized by the actions of selecting, rejecting, positioning, choosing, deciding, changing, wandering about, and looking deeper into that which one desires. The patient's gaze encounters that which it is creating, directing the production process, and enriching the end result.

It is important to pay attention to the techniques based on schools of psychology that are used in video art therapy workshops. Some of the elements which should be considered in the design and analysis of sessions are as follows:

- The reconstruction of reality: remake situations particularly at the stage of editing, when patients are able to reconstruct that reality symbolically.
- The construction of the symbolic world—desires, dreams, imagination, and memories—using the medium of video.
- The way contact is made and broken: getting in touch with the images made and also getting away from them.
- The integration of the four centers of the human being: body, mind, emotions, and spirit.

According to this, the "gaze" can be conceived as the driving force of the process: this has been confirmed in the description and analysis of practice. It is essential to pay attention to the position from which each participant views the process, as well as addressing what they choose to focus on. One must take into account the gaze of both the patient *and* the video art therapist, and the view which each takes of the production.

Video Art Therapy Practice

The best gift we can give others is to help them find their own power.
— (Marquier, 2000, p. 499)

Case Study 1

Six individual workshops, 2009. Urban context, in an association (day center), four female and two male adults with cerebral palsy, practice carried out with individuals. Type of practice: video workshop.

Case Study 2

Twenty-five individual sessions with supervision, 2011. Urban context, in an association (day center), 1 female adult with cerebral palsy, 50 hours of practice, 10 hours of supervision. Type of practice: video art therapy sessions.

Case Study 3

Nine group sessions with supervision, 2012–2015. Change of location for each session, a group of 7 participants, 36 hours of practice, 8 hours of supervision. Type of practice: video art therapy workshops.

The intention during practice was to pay attention to how both perception and the "gaze" were involved in the therapy process and to explore how this role developed over the course of the sessions. This analysis was carried out through the lens of three psychological schools: Gestalt therapy, psychoanalysis, and holism.

Throughout the sessions, it was possible to observe how the patients' "gaze" involved them in the process. Viewing was a key stage in this process of engagement, when patients were confronted not with what they wanted or believed to have captured with the camera, but with what they had actually filmed. This was an emotional moment: patients came up against mistakes or dashed hopes, frustration, or the surprise of something unexpected but exciting. From this initial emotional reaction, when participants began to encounter memories and moments from patients' lives, a subsequent stage was reached when the patient accepted the images generated as their own, and in this way became engaged in the process.

Examining this moment of patient engagement further, one can appreciate how dealing with the whole technical procedure (including errors, difficulties with format, and similar problems) as an integral part of it allowed the process of exploration to begin, with the encounter of emotions and memories, the use of symbolic imagery, and the reconstruction of reality.

Another fundamental observation I made during practice, particularly when working with a group, was that each person needed a very different amount of time to deepen in their exploration. Time is a key element in the video art therapy process. Additionally, my analysis of the sessions revealed participants' interest in combining audiovisual language with writing, acting techniques, visual arts, and music. Participants used games as the basis of many of their proposals. The elements that kept people engaged the most in both one-on-one sessions and workshops were dressing up, making up stories and characters, and talking about memories and dreams.

The models developed for data collection and the analysis of the production enabled me and the participants to recognize topics which may have gone unnoticed during the sessions that we picked up and explored later. Distancing oneself from events, putting thoughts and impressions on paper in as descriptive a way as possible, being attentive during sessions, and using observations to inform supervision were all key factors in ensuring that I conducted the data collection and analysis process rigorously.

My analysis demonstrated that creative processes which involve video result in a development of the "gaze," or participants' ways of seeing and interacting with the world. Regarding these participants, the patient's view of what they have produced is what gives them insight into the process of transformation they are experiencing. However, only when the patient has gone through the entire therapeutic process is their way of viewing the world significantly expanded; at which point they set out on the path toward change.

Important Observations

In this section, I attempt to draw together the most important observations I collected during the sessions and workshops. I found that at many points the video art therapist became as much of a protagonist as the patient. This is a factor which differentiates art therapy practice from other expressive arts therapies: it provides insights not only into the development of the patient and their production but also into the growth of the art therapist.

Continuous personal work and supervision leads the video art therapist to understand that it is the patient who is in control of the process. This enables the therapist to position themselves appropriately while they support the patient: being there for them and acting as a representative of that person's way of viewing and directing the production process.

Because this process is such a personal one, it may not be necessary for the video art therapist to share or understand all of it, a fact that can sometimes be frustrating for them. Finding an appropriate stance during the sessions allows the therapist to watch and listen to the patient, putting their ego and any internal struggles aside.

It is also important that the art therapist carries out their intervention in the art form in which they have expertise and which they find personally engaging. Since the therapist has been through what it's like to work with this art form, they can put themselves in the patient's shoes and connect with them more deeply.

The video art therapist's ways of seeing and acting in the sessions are fundamental. The relationship between video art therapist and patient clearly has great influence over how they develop and transform what the patient films. The main way the therapist and patient communicate to each other is through the production and the "gaze" they use to guide the process. Art can sometimes help us express ourselves when words fail.

The proposals, focus, and development of each type of session I observed were widely varied, but I did note some common themes. First, there was evidence of a clear, renewed engagement with video art as a therapeutic tool, with the question of technique being integrated into sessions—this allowed participants to focus on their own creative process. Second, the form of expression enabled by video became a liberating tool, centered as it is on the reconstruction of reality, constructing a symbolic world, contact, withdrawal, and the integration of the four human centers as described above. This tool allowed participants to develop new ways of seeing reality and to express their discontent, discomfort, interests, and feelings more clearly.

The second case study—centered on individual sessions with "Claudia"—produced some of the most profound insights of all the participants I observed. It was possible to see how, as use of the camera was gradually integrated into proposals and we began to play with the mobility of Claudia's body; these filmed images were able to create new, vibrant stories from a seemingly everyday reality. Claudia's filmed material was in this way able to take her—and her imagination—into a new creative space. In this new space, where she was exposed to worlds in which she had little experience until that moment, Claudia was able to find new ways of understanding reality, and herself.

From this starting point of emotional expression, it was possible, in Claudia's case, to provide evidence of the potential of audiovisual language as a liberating means of expressing one's spirituality. The video was able to show Claudia's inner strength and all of the things that usually show up in the unconscious and the self as a whole.

One of the most important findings of this practice is the link between the video-making process and the four centers of the human being: body, emotion, intellect, and spirituality. This is because, while all of these are always present in participants, each stage of the creative process places particular emphasis on one center over the others.

During the first stage of filming, corporality comes to the fore. Filming is the moment at which action commences. It is focused on the present moment, and all participants' energies are directed toward developing this action. The act of filming involves the whole body. In this part of the process, movement is the main character. Participants explore not only what they can feel with their senses, but also what they can see and change with their "gaze."

After filming, image and sound come to the foreground, when that which has been captured on film is viewed. The emotional center is predominant at this stage. During editing, cognition takes center stage. Editing allows the patient a chance to look into their imagination, their symbolic world, and their deepest desires.

The final part of the process is the analysis and further refinement of the film, when the time comes to take a new perspective and to choose between different paths. At this point, the focus is on transcendence and distancing oneself from authorship of the work. It is the ultimate goal of this type of therapy. It pays attention to the closure of sessions and to what happens afterward, understanding video as a tool for self-expression. The patients' "gaze" at this point is a holistic one that helps them think about themselves and the world around them.

Understanding the video production process in this way can help professionals to more clearly identify the aspects of the patient that they are working on at each stage of video art therapy sessions.

The most valuable aspect of video art therapy interventions is not the achievement of predetermined objectives. Instead, their most important contribution is the provision of alternatives and creative tools to help patients "rethink" themselves, the world around them, and the way they view themselves. Analysis of practice has shown that objectives do form part of the work proposed, even when a goal is not initially specified, but these aims are impossible to identify empirically. Rather, they can be appreciated by making observations from a phenomenological perspective. These objectives are oriented toward providing patients with the ability to reach a deeper understanding of themselves and giving them new perspectives from which to develop their internal world. From this point on, the aim is for patients to understand, accept, and relate to this internal reality and, finally, to be able to view the world from a new position.

Conclusion

In conclusion, the primary contribution of this observation and analysis of video art therapy has been to demonstrate the unique contribution of this practice to the art therapy field. It is important to pay attention to the means by which patient engagement is achieved and to how the process of transformation is realized, noting the great potential of combining video, art, and therapy as a tool for working with others. This tool can encourage patients to begin the process of developing self-awareness and bring them closer to a world that is constantly changing. The journey patients took over the course of the sessions, as they reached new levels of experience and understanding, serves as evidence that the widening of their "gaze"—their way of viewing and interacting with the world— opens up their world as a whole. What seems certain is that all new forms of reality that patients can envisage are worlds in which they will one day be able to live out their lives.

Notes

1 The term "gaze" has been used in this chapter in line with the concept's use in the fields of psychoanalysis, Gestalt psychotherapy and holism: more than just seeing the world, it is a way of both seeing, interpreting and directing action in the world. Given that the term is not used in English with the same frequency as its Spanish equivalent [*la mirada*], this term is mostly presented within quotation marks, but where "gaze" sounds least natural in English it has been substituted for "ways of seeing," "ways of seeing and acting," or "ways of viewing and directing."
2 "Production" is used throughout the chapter to refer to everything that patients produce in video art therapy sessions, including, but not limited to, that which becomes the finished product of a film.

References

Bergman, I. (1992). *Las mejores intenciones*) (Spanish Edition. Tusquets Editores.

Mampaso Martínez, A. (2001). *La video-animación: Aplicaciones en los campos del desarrollo social y comunitario, la educación artística y el arte terapia.* [Tesis doctoral, Universidad Complutense de Madrid].

Mampaso Martínez, A. (2004). Video-arte terapia y educación. In N. Martínez Díez & M. López Fernandez-Cao (Eds.), *Arteterapia y educación* (pp. 87–110). Comunidad de Madrid, Consejería de Educación. http://www.madrid.org/bvirtual/BVCM001479.pdf

Marquier, A. (2000). *La libertad de ser.* Ediciones Luciérnaga.

Rueda Cuenca, O. (2010). *La secuencia de cine como técnica en videoterapia.* DEA. Universidad Autónoma de Madrid.

Rueda Cuenca, O. (2018). *Videogestalt: Psicoterapia audiovisual (Vídeo, educación y terapia)* (Spanish Edition). Espaciointerno Ediciones.

13 Game Girls

Documentary Filmmaking and Drama Therapy Create the Potential Space of Self-Expression and Healing

Myriam D. Savage and Alina Skrzeszewska

Introduction

This chapter reviews and disseminates the unique documentary film and group support project called *Game Girls*, which marries the uses of documentary filmmaking with drama/expressive therapy for the benefit of sharing and healing the narratives of homeless women on Skid Row, Los Angeles, over a period of two years at the height of a growing population of destitute women in the area. The film won international accolades and awards, premiering at Berlinale Panorama, winning the Grand Jury Prize at FIFB in Bordeaux, France, and the CIMA award in Gijon, Spain, for the best feature directed by a woman. The film has played worldwide at over 30 festivals. During the film Q & As, audience members often shared their own trauma narratives of displacement and survival.

Six years later, the filmmaker and drama therapist delve into a reflective process with some of the participating women, covering the goals of the workshop and what one participant states is essential to all healing and creative processes, which is a responsible "follow-up" on the project's effects that invited a deep way of exploring themselves in a psychoeducational context and an active commitment to the filmed documentation of trauma in their lives. The documentary undoubtedly transformed the lives of those who invested in it: those who took part in its production and those who took part in being documented. Friendships grew and schisms occurred between strangers who shared intimately over a period of years. With the premise and understanding that real and vulnerable narratives were culled from our interactions in the group setting and during filming and even after its production, a committed group of us came together during a summer afternoon in 2020 to explore personal experiences with a follow-up aligned with the *potential* space of nurturing self-expression and healing in community (Winnicott, 1971) that is essential to healthy identity formation.

DOI: 10.4324/9781315622507-17

Project Context

In late 2013, a collaboration between registered drama therapist Myriam Savage, Ph.D., and documentary filmmaker Alina Skrzeszewska was forged when Alina reached out to Myriam about facilitating a drama therapy workshop for women on Skid Row, Los Angeles. The filmmaker had made previous documentary films there already and was interested in finding a new approach for this film that would be grounded in providing workshops to the growing community of homeless women in the area. In the fall of 2015, a state of emergency was declared for Skid Row. Its makeshift encampments on public sidewalks represented one of the largest areas of unsheltered people in the country; concentrated within a four-mile radius of downtown with more than 25,000 homeless in the city at the time, a quarter of them were part of a growing population of women. Seventy-five percent of homeless women sleep on the streets, and there has been a steady rise of women of all ages becoming homeless; anywhere from 36% to 40% of those women are victims of domestic abuse and mental illness as well as complex trauma, all of which are part of the overburdened landscape of Skid Row (Cabales, 2018). The filmmaker's goal was to create an opportunity for collaboration between the people behind and in front of the camera, as well as to provide a deeper experience for the audience who would eventually view the film that resulted from the workshops centered on therapeutic self-expression. To create a radically intimate documentary film about how and why women live on Los Angeles's infamous Skid Row, the filmmaker, producers, and registered drama therapist jointly created a free intensive weekly workshop for women in the neighborhood. Skrzeszewska aptly named the project *Game Girls*, as this seemed to best describe the conditions and machinations existing on Skid Row that the women had to manipulate and navigate to survive—a way of gaming systems involving social and health services, short-term shelters, long-term housing, and legal rights that drastically affect this population in downtown Los Angeles.

The Workshop Space for the Documentary

The filmmaking team secured a space from a supportive local downtown nonprofit organization, United Coalition East Prevention Project (UCEPP) for the workshop sessions that were situated in a storefront on Skid Row. UCEPP's work is centered in local drug prevention and community improvement efforts, and because it was established from the beginning that consistency and duration would be necessary for the success of the *Game Girls* workshops, having a set time and centralized place at UCEPP's location were essential to the success of offering our reliability for a mostly transient group. In 2014, the production team and drama therapist initially decided to meet twice a week, for three hours each day. In an environment such as Skid Row, where life is full of inconsistencies, the fact that this workshop would be available consistently each week provided a sense of safety and comfort for the participants. With the guidance of the drama therapist, the *Game Girls* staff and crew set up the room in a friendly and inviting way, with a colorful rug placed in the middle of a circle of chairs. The drama therapist brought other tools for art-making: fabrics, clay, masks, and acoustic instruments such as shakers for the action-based expressive arts group work. At each gathering, snacks and coffee were offered mid-session, and at the end. People struggle with profound poverty on Skid Row, and the belief was that many of the women came to depend on the healthy food provided (cheese, hummus, bread, veggie sticks, fruit, etc.). The women who attended workshops learned they shared commonality of childhood and complex trauma associated with domestic violence, addiction, self-harm, and the trauma of homelessness as well as intergenerational and historical harm. The majority of the group were women of color, with most identifying as Black or Latinx.

Participants in the Documentary

To recruit participants for the workshop, the filmmaking team canvassed the neighborhood with flyers. The filmmaker and producer reached out to case workers at local nonprofit organizations and to their own contacts from years of local involvement in the area. *Game Girls* invited people who identified as women to attend weekly support groups. All the while, the filmmaker's task of discovering the protagonists in the ensemble of participants occurred over a length of time. The finished film centered on the relationship and trauma of two women (Teri and Tiahna) from the ensemble. On January 31, 2014, the first workshop was launched in the storefront. Thirty women showed up and were asked why they considered attending the group. Some of the remarks documented then by the women who gave us permission to share their personal narratives without anonymity were as follows:

TERI: I was staying at an SRO [single room occupancy] building on Skid Row and there was a flyer. At the time I was going to Santa Monica College and taking a broadcasting class and what caught my eye was on the flyer.... And so I was like, all right, let me go check this out. Stay busy, do something positive in the community, instead of selling drugs or reverting back to my old ways or whatever. I felt it was a safe place for me to be at.

SILVIA: Safety is something that we all look for. To find a space where we feel comfortable, we don't feel judged, we can be ourselves, we can talk about our experiences without judgment. Because at the end [of the day], as women we've all been going through the same things, historically.

LORRAINE: …And when you talk about bipolar, I have it. And I try not to do the medication. I try to listen to people because I've been through a devastating life. […] Having bipolar, you need every force of energy that you can get to stay focused and not go crazy. You need these stepping stones. You need to be around people that believe in you, and who will help guide you in that direction, because it's not easy.

MARILYN: I wanted to do whatever I could to help other women in any way possible. So I told my story with the intention of being of service, with no agenda. Perhaps the reason is that I've been in recovery for over 30 years, and I learned a long time ago that to be of service really is what we're, as adults, encouraged to do.

Eventually, the group stabilized at around six to ten women per session, which was considered a great success rate for a program on Skid Row that didn't offer attendees any attached benefits for group therapy, such as signoffs on mandated counseling hours or a promise of accessing housing. After two months, the filmmaker and drama therapist decided to reduce workshop meetings to once a week, for three hours. With some breaks, these meetings continued until November 2015, and met sporadically afterward for extra sessions, reading performances and get-togethers, lasting for over two years of interaction before a documentary film was edited and produced for festival releases.

Drama Therapy on Skid Row

Drama therapy, a creative art therapy modality, which is standardized and accredited by the North American Drama Therapy Association (NADTA), is defined as the intentional use of theater arts and psychology for individuals or groups in clinical, educational, or community settings where the goal is facilitating emotional, psychological, cognitive, or physical needs of clients. In existence for over 40 years, its historical and psychodrama influences (Moreno, 1985) are evident in clinical, performance-based, and/or social justice-aimed implementations. Storytelling, role-playing, improvisation, performance, and projective techniques provided by art and mask work, metaphors, symbols, and theater rituals are drama therapy tools used in methods to reauthor problem-saturated self-narratives. The trained drama therapist is knowledgeable about trauma and creating opportunities for group members to utilize brave spaces where consensus is a driving force and where the work at hand is carefully paced through play and creativity while cultivating a safe place for emotional well-being.

Game Girls sessions were approached on a psycho-educational level due to several variables such as a lack of information to rely upon about the clinical diagnoses backgrounds of the weekly attendees because they were invited to participate right off the street through an open-door policy. With so many variables, groups were person-centered, informed by positive psychology (Fredrickson, 2001) and critical race feminist approaches (Mayor, 2012). Consent, waivers, and releases on film outcomes and participant responsibilities as well as confidentiality beyond the workshop were agreed upon between the drama therapy facilitator, participants, the director, and the production company. Dunne's (2006, 2009) *narradrama* method, a post-modern narrative therapy approach using embodied methods, influenced the action-based exercises and many of the interventions. The structure of the group workshops from onset to culmination was influenced by Emunah's (1994) Five Phases drama therapy method. Guest artists and colleagues such as Boal expert Mady Schutzman and playwright and continuum movement practitioner Jean Claude van Itallie guest-facilitated writing and acting workshops on Skid Row.

Throughout, participants experienced themselves and peers doing improvisation and role-playing resulting in gestalt-like experiences that were also verbally processed in the sessions. Pathologizing and labels around homelessness were to be replaced by personal agency. Psychologist/drama therapist Landy (1986, 1991) refers to agency in the impersonation of roles such as the hero's journey, a role recognized at the core of the middle phase of the project when a therapeutic public performance stemming from a Sylvia Plath poem ("The Mirror," 1971) spurred on an original play about the women's experiences with age and life changes (Plath, 1980). The arc of the weekly workshops began with phase one of community building, accessing a way to collaborate through improvisation and projective techniques, which led to a second phase within the first year of exploring and producing performance and deeper work on self-identity through making original self-masks and writing. This evolved to the final phase of the sessions focused on the celebration and acceptance of self-identity despite past life trauma experiences.

The Marriage of Documentary Filmmaking and Drama Therapy

Combining the two professions affected ways of interacting with participants within group dynamics. Gathering women together as an ensemble of witnesses to each other's personal stories while filming workshops became a route toward creating a community. The original intention of the *Game Girls* project was not about using filmmaking as a tool for therapy. The project was to utilize drama therapy in the workshop sessions, often heeding the filmic needs of the director and always following the lead of the participants on themes to address. The filmmaker documented actions and life inside and outside of the storefront. Drama therapy as well as documentary interview techniques that the filmmaker used invited sensitization to problematic personal, historical, socio-economic, systemic narratives. The added boon was the women's therapeutic experiences. The filmmaker was not set on a plan for how the film would be edited, for instance. Women were invited to explore life stories in an albeit unconventional way while film cameras and boom operators existed in the room. After a while, the technical crew's existence was normalized. Initially, new group members would "play to the camera" until prompted to ignore it during improvisational games and other group actions, which they eventually did with ease. Their explored and re-storied lived and fictional narratives increasingly became more the focus of the group gatherings. As a result, the film audience views snippets of the therapeutic space of play and creativity in the finished film, featured in the short scenes of the storefront sessions, showing the women processing drama therapy methods facilitated by the therapist.

Though the film primarily chronicles the relationship between two women dealing with the adverse effects of mental illness, addiction, and social systems set up to support those on disability, those adversities were familiar experiences for all the women involved. Hardships shared between the two protagonists who experienced complex trauma predominate the film's narrative. Mutual aid and a strength-based ideology (Shulman, 2011) about resiliency were foundational for finding common ground through the experiential exercises and discussions in the therapeutic space.

The Film Camera as a Therapeutic Tool

Halverson (2010) posited that "identity is concretized through the narratives we tell of our own lives" (p. 2355). Her research invited young participants to make original, autobiographical video narratives which "demonstrated that it is through the process of telling, adapting, and performing narratives of personal experience that adolescents engage in positive identity development" (p. 2356)—an argument that could apply to the experiences of older women facing complex trauma. Johnson and Alderson (2008) researched therapeutic filmmaking involving three counseling clients (aged late 20s) making and discussing short films they shot about personal experiences (p. 11), which resulted in client empowerment. Before the digital age, Hoorwitz (1984) noted video therapy with young participants watching themselves role-play about family difficulties held positive effects, de-synthesizing problem-saturated narratives.

Witnessing the Self on Film

Richert's (2003) point that "self is understood as both story and the process of storying" (p. 208) was a lived result of *Game Girls* through the revelation that Irwin (1977) unpacks for us: the drama of explored life is played out through the experiential, therapeutic process. This and Richert's (2003) narrative theory that exploring personal story occurs in the interaction with others are evident in those inserted film snippets when personal stories of marginalization and trauma are processed in the miniature worlds the women create. Yet, when the filmmaker presented early workshop outtakes, some participants found it difficult to view themselves on screen and a few decided to discontinue attending. Similarly, Hinz and Ragsdell's (1990) intentional use of video for self-identity research with women who had bulimia resulted in several participants not willing to show up to sessions once they viewed themselves on screen.

At the advent of video therapy usage, McNiff and Cook (1975) devised a two-year art therapy study using video playback and visual portrait-making with clients who had behavioral issues from mental illness, inviting them to videotape, edit, and view film documenting their spontaneous interactions in art-making sessions, which resulted in cathartic responses adjusting behavior, self-evaluation, and communication. Novy (2003) supported hospitalized adolescent participants in a study where they wrote, directed, and acted in a video that was based on fictional and metaphorical characters. They were able to separate from identified problems and fixed identities of mental illness through a private video viewing of their original film. Savage (2016, 2018, 2019) utilized digital visual apps in narrative research with young women adopted from foster care, noting that privately viewing their recorded mock personal public service announcements (PPSAs) featuring their preferred resilient identities opened up conversations about personal histories even after they chose to publicly watch the PPSAs with support systems. Orr (2005, 2006) concludes that therapists using digital video media must account for the "inherent qualities of the medium" (p. 1) and consider the clients' therapeutic processes and needs. While technology offers adaptive tools, it still requires training to adhere to best practices.

Discussion

Apprehending the Self

Overlapping multiple media and their approaches may enhance and increase participation and interests in people (Barone & Eisner, 2012), which was evident in *Game Girls* workshops as various modes of exploration and media used for self-expression increased. During the second phase of workshops, the camera was implemented as a role-playing tool with the original self-masks and costumes the women created. The drama therapist invited participants to identify with the dual internal and external roles depicted in their self-masks and to speak directly to the camera, which resulted in self-revelation and unpacking trauma experiences. This was an example of overlapping media and approaches exemplifying Novy's (2003) theory that a healthy separate identity evolves in film work with drama therapy when participants are compelled to "apprehend" (Irwin, 1977, p. 428) themselves from some other perspective. The use of masks gave an added protection on film as well as a preferred self-image that was presented in this exercise—a way to face themselves through the images they created (Dunn-Snow & Joy-Smellie, 2000; Savage, 2016, 2018, 2019).

Ultimately, the filmed segment of the exercise was not included in the final cut, but Landy's (1986, 1991) point that role-playing is central to dramatic experience and to gaining perspective could be argued as central to such an exercise and in the therapeutic theater production (*Rock/Paper/Scissors*) that consequently ensued. Cattanach (1994) posits that the role-taker assimilates two realities of "the everyday and the fictional[,] imaginatively holding them in paradoxical relationship to one another" (p. 23), which is what filmed participants eventually disclose about the overall workshop experience in the ensuing follow-up and what the audience witnesses when viewing the documentary, allowing them to see the everyday reality of Skid Row on the outside of the group setting and the imaginary, therapeutic play encouraged within it.

Follow-Up

Participants in the *Game Girls* project lacked control over their own narratives that were being filmed, and the sense of empowerment from hands-on filming was not part of their experience as it was for others in a therapeutic sense (Halverson, 2010; Hoorwitz, 1984; Johnson & Alderson, 2008; McNiff & Cook, 1975; Novy, 2003; Savage, 2016, 2018, 2019); this even becomes a point of serious concern, as is evident from the participants' disclosures included below. The *Game Girls* project did not offer digital or video story-making solutions for self-expression because this was never the intent. Six years later, we follow up as a core collective and offer up the opportunity to understand the evolving effects of the *Game Girls* experience with the following excerpts of dialogue we are permitted to share about the collaboration with the film camera and drama therapy:

On the Filmmaking Process

SILVIA: The camera..., when you're not used to it, it feels funny, awkward, and I realized it changes the behavior of people. It changes the behavior when you're aware or too aware. [...] I've never been too confident with pictures or something where I can see myself. I feel weird, awkward. I say, "Oh, Silvia, what are you doing there? You didn't fix your hair."

TERI: I would completely forget! I would get nervous when I'm getting mic'd up but then after that, I'll forget.

SYLVIA: If they are going to take a picture of me, I hope they give me the best angles.

TERI: I don't know my best angles!

SYLVIA: The ego just blooms.

Reactions and Reflection about the Film

TERI: I was embarrassed at first. Because it [the workshop] was about all of us, you know what I mean? A lot of stories that was shared. That's what I anticipated on seeing. And so I was a little shocked that it [the movie] was centered around me and Tiahna. I mean, it felt good a little bit. Like, who doesn't want a film about them? You know, it feels good a little bit, but at the same time I like being behind the scenes. I don't like to be on the forefront.

MARILYN: Now, I personally, as we continued with this, I did have ideas of what it was going to be, how it was going to be presented and that's not what happened.

SILVIA: I didn't really know, but I thought it [the film] would be related with the workshops. And I was disappointed when I saw the movie about the relationship. [...] Skid Row has been a place of coming and taking, that's why. In the [inaudible 00:20:20] that is being created around any narratives and the expectations. So that's why I was concerned because when I saw that [the movie] I saw sensationalism, what it can sell, what it reach out to more people, of people that expect from Skid Row downtown.

LORRAINE: When I saw this movie, I thought it was excellent. I thought it [...] showed that women had to stick together because men was not there for them. With the relationship, you guys are showing that this is what goes on for real. And then when we're in the group [inside the workshop], that's the background. That's why you was in the group because your head was going to another way and you needed to calm down. A relationship is going to be at a crossfire no matter where you are. But on Skid Row, it's impossible to even have a relationship. [...] I was in Skid Row in the 80s, and actually, it just started being Skid Row, really bad, people really becoming homeless in the 80s. I ended up sleeping in a doorway for eight years. So I know. Fred Jordan had me on TV talking about what was going on downtown and I talked about the women and how they was being treated and stuff like that. I was shot, stabbed, raped. Fought for my life because I knew my parents did not teach me to be eating out no damn trashcan. [...] And so all the women saw it, the guys, well, they saw it on the news and all the women be crossing the street [to talk to me]. And they said, thank you so much for what you said. Because no one had put it out there like that. [...] I am so grateful that I could be a wonderful example for people. And that's what it's all about. It's not easy because people are going to have their opinions about you. But I don't care because I could've been dead.

TERI: Some people told me it was too hard for them to watch because they didn't want to see me in that situation.

MARILYN: I would like it [the movie] to show more of the different storylines and the drama therapy actions that we took. [...] One of the days a friend of mine died. And I came in [to the workshop] anyway. I went through appendicitis. I came in anyway. I had kidney stones and I came in anyway. The perseverance, the determination. So things like that, that's what I would like to see.

SILVIA: I just appreciated this space and getting to know others, and I was longing to go there and do art and I was excited with the performance, all the activities, all that we were doing together. For me, that was the richest part of the project.

What You Got Out of the Workshop Project

LORRAINE: Everybody was so present, not fussing or anything. It looked like everybody wanted to be released of the pain that was going inside of them. And we was in the comfort zone to make that happen.

TERI: It's like once we was there in the workshops, even though it was downtown Skid Row, it didn't feel like we was downtown Skid Row. It felt like we were somewhere else for those moments. And then everybody was just [...] It's like we knew each other already. Once we were there, everybody left everything at the door and we were happy to be [...] I was happy. I can speak for myself. I was happy to be in a room with women where we all just had our guard down and we were there for each other for moral support, regardless of what the other person was talking about. We were there to support one another and be there for one another. So that's what kept me going and sticking with it. It was a safe place and it was fun. And I love the hummus.

MARILYN: It was more of my heart and soul opening up, becoming even more empathetic. I'd been a homeless advocate. I was again homeless in my life. And I was getting the understanding that I wasn't alone, that all these other people who I'd not met in my life had similar experiences of abuse, disassociation, homelessness, by really nothing I did. It wasn't anything that I did that I became homeless.

TERI: I felt alone until I came to the workshops. I was happy to go to the workshops. I was like, I'm going to the group. Be with my peers. It was very, very comforting. Like I said, it was a world away from [...] I wasn't on Skid Row.

MARILYN: It was a sanctuary. [All agree.] It was a safe place [...] even though there's always going to be difference of opinions. People are going to take things wrong. That's always going to happen whenever you have people together.

SILVIA: That's the beauty of it, no? We are all different. We have different points of view.

MARILYN: You grow by experiencing other people's concepts and having a facilitator with the skills to be able to bring it in to a safe place again. To command respect for each other, regardless of what you believe or feel.

SILVIA: I feel like you said, you have to be willing, open minded. When you realize, it's okay to be here. You start caring for people. You find people that you connect with, and you make relationships. Build these relationships and nourish them. That was one of the parts that brought me to a bigger spectrum of trust. I'm safe too. I can trust. What I grasped from that experience, I've been putting it into use. I've been having the opportunity to be in so many spaces in that sense. Okay, you just blending, and you just throw in this formation and putting us together. It's been so valuable for me.

ALINA (FILMMAKER): One thing that I wanted to ask you Silvia specifically though, is because I remember you talking in the workshops about relationships with women, not trusting women. Now you're talking about wanting to do stuff with women.

SYLVIA: Thank you very much. That's why I appreciated the workshop because that was a growing process for me. To understand that we can trust each other. I learned that I was sensing that, but I learned eventually that it wasn't a unique feeling. I learned that a lot of us—we have that because we are so proud to emulate these patriarchal roles. All of us, a lot of us, we have that. That sense of authority or that "we want to have this," be the boss or whatever. Because it's emulating these patriarchal roles. Now I understand it and now I feel I'm better and now I'm learning how to manage it. It's great. The growth for me is huge because [of] the work that I started doing in the community, and what's important for me too. You have to, like—release yourself from those layers of whatever you want to call them. They are bothering you. There's a burden. It doesn't allow you to move forward in your growth.

TERI: The workshops really did help me and Tiahna. I remember in the film, she said, she's blooming. She's growing now. I think you asked her, what did she mean by that? She couldn't really explain it, but I noticed that the workshops would serve a great purpose for her because she didn't have that community type of thing. I was more raised on love. She was more raised on survival. When she came to the workshops, I saw that she was able to see a different part of herself. And she's been different ever since then. Even though we're not together, we co-parent amazingly. I keep the boy all the time. [...] But even though [...] we're not in a relationship, it's crazy because we have a better friendship. She trusted me to take him when he was one years old, to Shreveport, Louisiana, to see my family. I took him on his first plane. I teach him how to use his potty. I teach him how to tie his shoes. I teach him everything, all his first things. She's given me the opportunity to do that. Thank you. And I love it. I'm so excited. Like the fact that we're not together, but the fact that I'm able to grow with him, man it's amazing.

SILVIA: One thing that I learned about programs from wherever county, city, local, grassroots, whatever, whoever, if we don't follow up, that sense of, like, feeling of hope or connectedness is going to fade. That's what I learned. Anything that we can, we could start, it has to have a follow-up.

Conclusion

White (1995, 2000) argues that witnessed reflection prevalent in this method of narrative-based workshopping and even in the above follow-up may provide a ceremony important to positive identity formation and a tangible way to strategize against being marginalized. These processes may improve interpersonal and intrapersonal needs for anyone working in a creative ensemble. Glăveanu (2011) describes how trust and a feeling of safety for group members takes place in a *representational* space or else "the risk of exposing ideas or engaging with the ideas of others" (p. 485) preempts engagement. He refers to Winnicott's (1971) *potential* space in developmental theory with this observation—a third place borne of cultural experience located between individuals and the environment (p. 135)—an area of new experiences, of play shaped by ever-changing social interactions. This *potential* space existed during the *Game Girls* encounter; within a storefront, via the life of the documentary and in this follow-up as we create the communal encounter for more self-expression. Considering these collaboration theories, we wonder if the careful use of the camera lens helps to further secure the *potential* third space of trust and safety for marginalized voices while we deem that documentary filmmaking with drama therapy enhances the therapeutic aims of group dynamics, validating underrepresented voices (Figures 13.1–13.6).

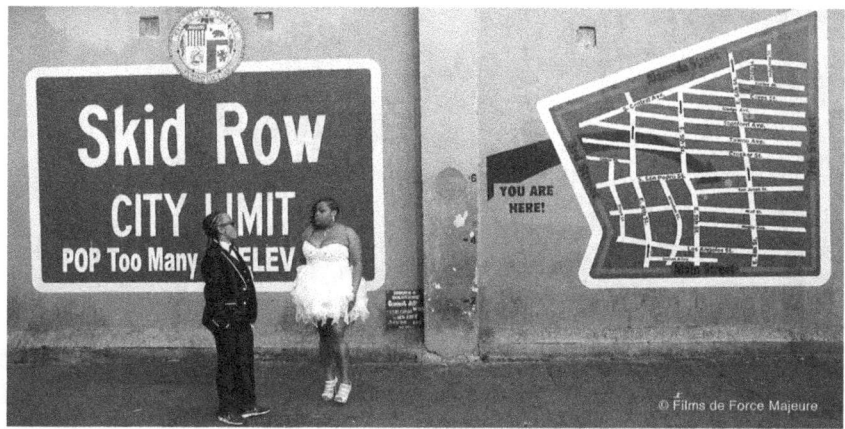

Figure 13.1 Game Girls film protagonists Teri and Tiahna on Skid Row.

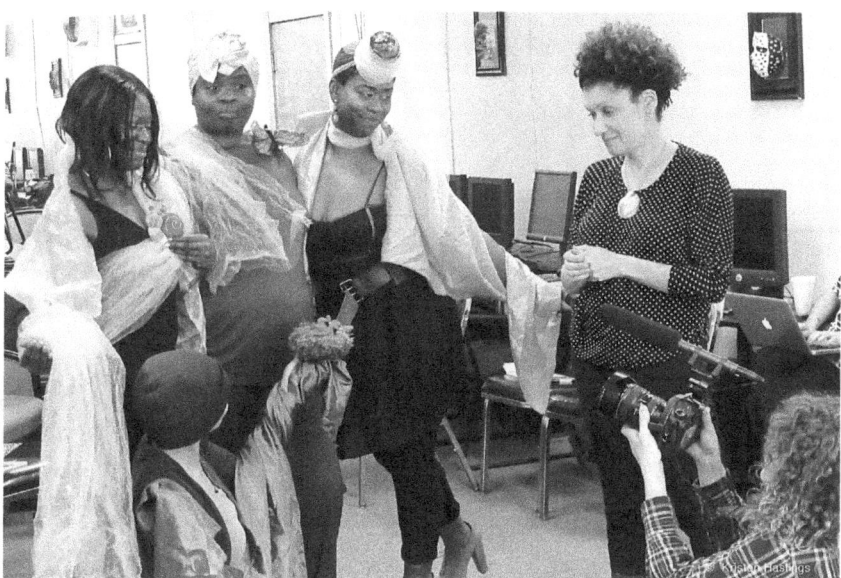

Figure 13.2 Filming drama therapy group with drama therapist in storefront, Skid Row.

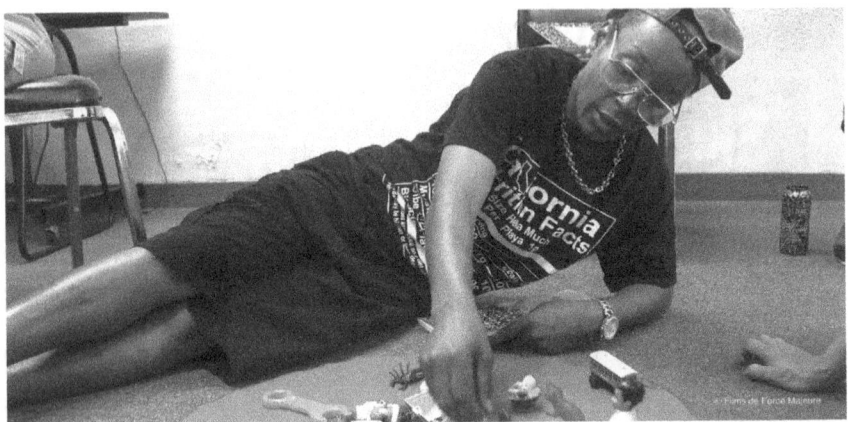

Figure 13.3 Facilitating projective methods with Teri during Game Girls group workshop.

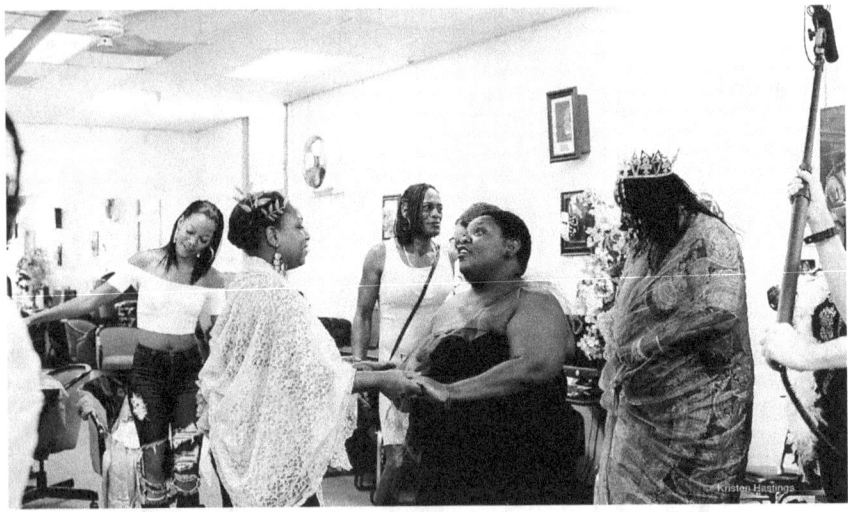

Figure 13.4 Game Girls drama therapy celebratory workshop on self-identity.

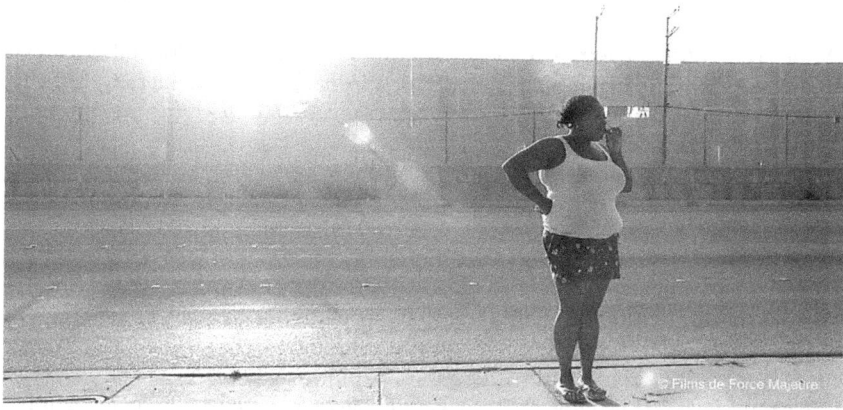

Figure 13.5 Film protagonist Tiahna waiting for Teri's release from county jail.

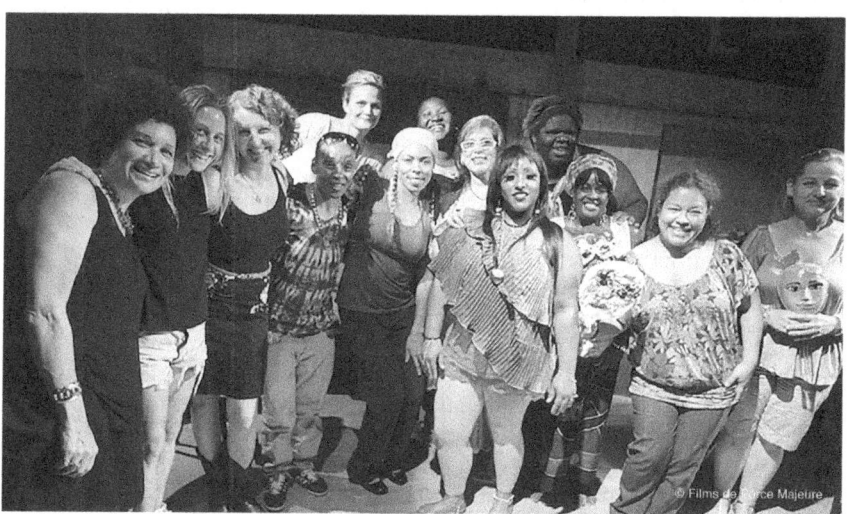

Figure 13.6 Game Girls project cast, crew, film director, drama therapist from Rock/Paper/Scissors therapeutic theatre performance.

References

Barone, T., & Eisner, E. W. (2012). *Arts based research*. SAGE. doi: 10.4135/9781452230627

Cabales, V. (2018). Homeless in California—What the data reveals. Retrieved from https://calmatters.org/housing/2018/06/homeless-in-california-what-the-data-reveals/

Cattanach, A. (1994). *Play therapy: Where the sky meets the underworld.* Jessica Kingsley.

Dunne, P. (2006). *The narrative therapist and the arts* (2nd ed.). Possibilities Press.

Dunne, P. (2009). Narradrama: A narrative approach to drama therapy. In D. R. Johnson & R. Emunah (Eds.), *Current approaches in drama therapy* (pp. 172–204). Charles C. Thomas.

Dunn-Snow, P., & Joy-Smellie, S. (2000). Teaching art therapy techniques: Mask-making, a case in point. *Art Therapy: Journal of the American Art Therapy Association, 17*(2), 125–131. doi: 10.1080/07421656.2000.10129512

Emunah, R. (1994). *Acting for real: Drama therapy process, technique, and performance.* Routledge.

Fredrickson, B. L. (2001). The role of positive emotions in positive psychology: The broaden-and-build theory of positive emotions. *American Psychologist, 56*(3), 218–226. doi: 10.1037/0003-066X.56.3.218

Glăveanu, V.-P. (2011). How are we creative together? Comparing sociocognitive and sociocultural answers. *Theory and Psychology, 21*(4), 473–492. doi: 10.1177/0959354310372152

Halverson, E. R. (2010). Film as identity exploration: A multimodal analysis of youth-produced films. *Teachers College Record, 112*(9), 2352–2378. doi: 10.1177/016146811011200903

Hinz, L. D., & Ragsdell, V. (1990). Using masks and video in group psychotherapy with bulimics. *The Arts in Psychotherapy, 17*(3), 259–261. doi: 10.1300/J182v02n02_13

Hoorwitz, A. N. (1984). Videotherapy in the context of group therapy for late-latency children of divorce, *Psychotherapy Journal 12*(1), 48–53. https://doi.org/10.1037/h0087528

Irwin, E. (1977). Play, fantasy, and symbols: Drama with emotionally disturbed children. *American Journal of Psychotherapy, 31*, 426–436. doi: 10.1176/appi.psychotherapy.1977.31.3.426

Johnson, J. L., & Alderson, K. G. (2008). Therapeutic filmmaking: An exploratory pilot study. *The Arts and Psychotherapy, 35*, 11–19. doi: 10.1016/j.aip.2007.08.004

Landy, R. J. (1986). *Drama therapy: Concepts and practices.* Charles C. Thomas.

Landy, R. J. (1991). Role as the primary bridge between theatre and drama therapy. *Dramatherapy, 13*(1), 4–11. doi: 10.1080/02630672.1991.9689795

Mayor, C. (2012). Playing with race: A theoretical framework and approach for creative arts therapists, *The Arts in Psychotherapy, 39*(3), 214–219. doi: 10.1016/j.aip.2011.12.008

McNiff, S., & Cook, C. (1975). Video art therapy. *The Arts in Psychotherapy 2*(1), 55–63. doi: 10.1016/0090-9092(75)90027-7

Moreno, J. L. (1985). *Psychodrama: First volume.* Beacon House.

Novy, C. (2003). Drama therapy with pre-adolescents: A narrative perspective. *The Arts in Psychotherapy, 30*, 201–207. doi: 10.1016/S0197-4556(03)00055-8

Orr, P. P. (2005). Technology media: An exploration for "inherent qualities". *The Arts in Psychotherapy, 32*, 1–11. doi: 10.1016/j.aip.2004.12.003

Orr, P. P. (2006). Technology training for art therapists: Is there a need? *Art Therapy: Journal of the American Art Therapy Association, 23*(4), 191–196. doi: 10.1080/07421656.2006.10129329

Plath, S. (1980). *Crossing the water*. Harper Perennial.

Richert, A. (2003). Living stories, telling stories, changing stories. Experiential use of the relationship in narrative therapy. *Journal of Psychotherapy Integration, 13*(2), 188–210. doi: 10.1037/1053-0479.13.2.188

Savage, M. (2018). Young women adopted from foster care create personal public service announcements: Narrative constructs in arts-based enquiry. *Qualitative Research in Psychology, 17*(2), 204–221. doi: 10.1080/14780887.2018.1442692

Savage, M. D. (2016). Listening to the voices of young women adopted from foster care through personal public service announcements. *Drama Therapy Review, 2*(2), 195–209. doi: 10.1386/dtr.2.2.195_1

Savage, M. D. (2019). Personal public service announcements: Collaborating with young women adopted from foster care using narradrama and an iPad during arts-based narrative inquiry. In I. R. Berson, M. J. Berson, & Gray, C. (Eds.), *Research in global child advocacy, Vol. 7: Participatory methodologies to elevate children's voices and agency* (pp. 203–227). Information Age.

Shulman, L. (2011). *The dynamics and skills of group counseling*. Brooks/Cole.

White, M. (1995). *Re-authoring lives: Interviews and essays*. Dulwich Centre Publications. Retrieved from http://www.narrativetherapylibrary.com/free-

White, M. (2000). *Reflections on narrative practice: Essays and interviews*. Dulwich Centre Publications. Retrieved from http://www.dulwichcentre.com.au/articles-about-narrative-therapy.html

Winnicott, D. W. (1971). *Playing and reality*. Routledge.

14 Producing a Documentary as a Therapeutic Process for Victims of Childhood Sexual Abuse

Yarden Kerem

Introduction

It is generally accepted that the documentary is a film genre intended to document reality. Bill Nichols, a theorist, critic, and documentary film researcher, writes that the power of documentary films lies in directing our gaze to matters that need attention and observation. The documentary explores social issues, events, problems, and suggested solutions (Nichols, 2001, p. 2). While watching a documentary, viewers expect it to describe an existing reality, while also expecting authenticity (Nichols, 2001, pp. 6–7).

Michael Renov, a film lecturer and film researcher, proposes that the documentary film has four roles:

A   To document, discover, and preserve
B   To promote an idea
C   To analyze or investigate
D   To be a tool of expression

(Renov, 1993, p. 21)

In this chapter, I offer another role of documentary cinema: as a therapeutic tool for its creator. That is, the documentary has an additional role beyond the four roles that Renov proposed, and Nichols's assertion that cinema is for exploring social issues. Furthermore, I contend that filmmakers who are survivors of childhood sexual abuse have three uniquely interwoven identities: director, film creator, and assault victim. These identities, or personas, add to the complexity of making a personal documentary.

When a trauma victim decides to produce a personal film about their assault, from the moment they have made up their mind to do so to the moment the movie is screened and an interaction is formed with the audience watching the film, the victim goes through a healing process from which they benefit. This healing occurs during the filmmaking process, for the following reasons:

DOI: 10.4324/9781315622507-18

1 Making documentary films obligates the filmmaker to form a narrative: the maker must first tell who he was before the assault, define the type of the assault, and explain the impacts of this assault and how that person lived their life following it. The healing process is one of transformation from traumatic memory to a narratorial one (Deshe, 2017, p. 74). Therefore, the very creation of a narrative is a healing process.

2 Testimony: the film allows its director to provide a testimony of their life. Theories and diverse therapeutic approaches have dealt with one's testimony of their situation. This testimony allows the testifier to receive recognition from her peers as a therapeutic act, just as Cathy Caruth (1996), Shoshana Felman and Dori Laub (2008)

3 The therapeutic perception of Wilfred Bion concerns the creation of a vessel that can contain difficult content, on the transference of Alpha materials to Beta ones, reverie, and the projective identification (see Bell, 2008). Film contains these therapeutic elements.

4 Film contains multiple elements of Winnicott's therapeutic perception: therapy as a game, the in-between space, feeling omnipotence, and the concept of Holding (see Winnicott, 2010a).

5 Film contains elements of Ogden's therapeutic perception: dream space, the analytic third (Ogden, 2013).

6 Visibility as a therapeutic tool: visibility; one who can see himself (in the mirror, in the stills, or on the screen), addressing another person, who sees himself, is a central part of the therapeutic process occurring while making a personal film. Visibility appears in literary scholarship by many acknowledged theoreticians, such as Freud, Kohut, Lacan, and Winnicott. Film contains multiple elements of Kohut's therapeutic perception: empathy, self-cohesion, self-object, and transmuting internalization (Kohut, 2005).

7 Group dynamics: the group dynamics has been a recognized therapeutic method since the 1940s. Since a gathering of two people constitutes a group, I find that joint work on a personal film contains therapeutic values fitting a group dynamic: mostly, the element which Yalom dubbed *cohesiveness* (Yalom and Leszcz, 2006, pp. 72–80).

8 Films that have to do with trauma incorporate healing elements, in accordance with methods that deal with therapy through art (Malchiodi, 2011): self-expression, active participation, imagination, and body-mind relation. Finally, healing from trauma requires a person to tackle three significant barriers: the recovery paradox, the need for revenge, and the attack on hope.

I wrote this chapter after viewing three documentary films produced in Israel by directors who testified in their films that they were victims of sexual abuse as children: *The Diamond Inside* (Keren Lev-Muhrberg, 1998), *Pursued* (Menachem Roth, 2012), and *Dirty Laundry* (Yael Scherer, 2012).

Even if the directors had studied cinema, this was the first film each of them produced. They were previously unknown in the world of cinema. I found that these directors did not follow the theory of Paula Rabinowitz, the film researcher. Rabinowitz (1994) opined that documentary films express the voices of minorities and excluded audiences; the documentary carries their voices because they cannot speak for themselves (p. 12). This chapter points to films in which excluded minorities—in this case, victims of acute trauma—have taken it upon themselves to make their own voices heard, despite a lack of power and authority. That is, the minority—the individual, the injured person—found a way to recount not only what happened to them, but to do so through a process that encourages, promotes, and brings about healing.

In this chapter, I assume that producing a personal documentary is a therapeutic process. I assume the therapeutic process that accompanied the filmmaking was the goal, or one of the goals, of producing the film, whether that motivation was a clear and conscious choice of the director or not. Because readers will not have access to these films, I do not discuss the films themselves in depth, but reflect my understanding of documentary cinema as a therapeutic tool for trauma situations in general, and trauma from sexual abuse in particular. I find that the documentary contains some very important and intriguing healing elements for victims of this type of trauma.

Film Production as a Therapeutic Event

Judith Lewis Herman writes that trauma victims lose a sense of control over their lives. They lose a sense of connection and meaning. Traumatic events cause profound and long-term changes in the body, emotions, consciousness, and memory. These functions that are usually intertwined may detach from one another following the trauma. Traumatic symptoms have a tendency to break away from their source and have a life of their own. Trauma victims feel and act as if their nervous system has been cut off from the present. They have no ability to defend themselves.

The many symptoms of post-traumatic stress disorder are divided into three main categories: over-excitation, invasion, and reduction:

- Over-excitation: Reflects the constant expectation of danger
- Invasion: Reflects the unmistakable seal of the traumatic moment
- Reduction: Reflects the blurring response of submission

(Herman, 2011, pp. 50–51)

Sexual injury inflicts a severe experience of helplessness and loss of control. The act of producing the film, and even the final product of the film itself, serves an anchor of control for the creator. What was a devastating experience becomes not only a testimony of the event but also a healing testimony.

Yael Deshe writes about the experience of sexual trauma of an abused child as a trauma that begins without words, without memory, without symbolic representations. The sexual trauma experience is an occurrence without continuity and order; in many cases, it is subconscious. It is an experience recorded in the body and the senses, but as fragments of unrelated, dark, secret feelings. The experience of sexual harm is a horror that creates paralysis and speechlessness and cannot be physically and mentally contained. It's an unthinkable experience. The threat to physical and psychological perfection produces helplessness and horror. The secret and the silence create displacement from a previous existence, a displacement that leaves the child detached from reality and the unknown (Deshe, 2017, pp. 70–71).

In this chapter, I propose that during the production of a personal documentary about sexual injury, the director is reacquainted with these difficulties—an experience of disconnected sensations, paralytic and mute, an experience that the body and mind cannot accept—that require the director to cope with all these conflicting elements. The victim's nervous system is unstable and damaged, and although the experience is chaotic and sometimes wordless, the tendency after trauma is to stay silenced and to self-isolate. In direct contradiction, producing the film requires the director to be forthcoming as the source of all the conflict created by the trauma, thus paving the way for healing herself.

Healing Elements Inherent in Documentary Cinema

I suggest the following eight healing elements are inherently found in documentary cinema.

1   Recovery Through the Construction of the Narrative

Tuval-Mashiach and Patton (2019) state, "The traumatic memories remain isolated and uncorrelated with the rest of the autobiographical memories, which often leads to non-adaptive self-perceptions of the event" (p. 239). Yael Deshe writes that the recovery process can take place "only in a relationship where a transformation from traumatic memory to narrative memory occurs" (Deshe, 2017, p. 78). Furthermore, "The rebuilding of the traumatic experience restores the process of testimony that collapsed during the abuse" (Deshe, 2017, pp. 82–83). The therapeutic goal is to allow the patient to tell the traumatic story in a coherent way, with sequence and meaning. A movie requires the construction of a new sequential narrative.

Human memory is encoded in two paths: one is encoding verbally accessible knowledge. This knowledge, as Tuval-Mashiach and Patton explain, is associated with conscious autobiographical memories: the patient is aware of them and remembers them and can verbalize them.

The second path is a less-conscious, nonverbal track, connected to the senses and unconscious channels (situationally accessible knowledge). Treatment, according to the narrative and other models, requires the trauma patient to combine the processing of the two memory pathways. Such treatment should address "both the construction of the conscious, literal narrative that involves the construction and restoration of impaired cognitions and meanings, and to aspects encoded in the implicit sensory memory, which involve physical and sensory responses" (Tuval-Mashiach & Patton, 2019, p. 240). Cinema allows for a combination of the two pathways, as it allows the creation of a verbal narrative alongside experiential work with nonverbal sensory characteristics.

2   Testimony as a Therapeutic Event

To create a film, the director has to give evidence of what he has been through. He has to come out of the paralysis and break the silence in order to create. He must connect the pieces of the experiences to a coherent and continuous narrative that has a beginning, a middle and an end. Yael Deshe writes that losing one's ability to witness oneself is the true meaning of self-extinction that occurs during sexual assault (Deshe, 2017, p. 78). Losing the ability to be your own witness disturbs your ability to think and understand yourself, impairing the ability to construct a coherent and meaningful life narrative while also weakening the ability to verbalize the experience. The director of the film is obliged to rescue/extract herself from the state of collapse of her own testimony about her life—from the state of not knowing the trauma—to a neat and contained story of the trauma.

The most significant thing that happens during the therapy of filmmaking is bearing witness to what actually happened. Giving testimony in front of another person is not a personal, internal process. The testimony is the victim knowing that there is at least one other person witnessing his injury. Giving testimony is a process in which one understands and learns about oneself. In a chapter titled "Bearing Witness, or the Vicissitudes of Listening," Dori Laub writes that the realization and knowledge of the event only occurs once the person who has been traumatized tells the story. Giving testimony is a process that involves the listener. Therefore, the listener has a significant part in creating the knowledge. The one listening to the trauma, for a moment, becomes enmeshed in the traumatic event by vicariously sharing and reliving it. The testimony changes something for the listener and the speaker (Felman & Laub, p. 67). The truth is revealed through this process.

The testimony is like reclaiming the event. Once the testimony is given, there is a deep sense of liberation. The testimony is liberating and vital.

The film provides evidence of a crisis. Viewers of the film take part in the traumatic event and are partners in accepting it. They experience the trauma, even if it is only in a partial manner. The testimony is the externalization of the event in order for it to be processed, so it can then be brought back in, to further process it.

Laub emphasizes the need for an audience to listen to the narrative as *active* listeners. A listener who experiences the event processes and adapts it. Laub's ideas can be more deeply understood through Bion's explanation of the concept of projective identification.

3   Projective Identification in Cinema: Wilfred Bion's Theory

Freud said unwanted parts of our selves are thrown out. Feelings within the person are split and are projected outward. The projection outward means we assume it is happening to someone else. The person experiences the emotions outside of herself. Melanie Klein has renewed and added the concept of Projective Identification: the parts actually move and live externally in the object, but there is something in the person which continues to be connected to and identify with the parts of herself that she projected outwards. The baby that projects onto her mother put parts of herself in her mother and then experiences them returning to her through her mother.

The Projection Identification mechanism is a complex operation: when the person projects outward, he is still connected to the parts he has projected outward. They are still part of the Self. It is a mechanism for releasing anxieties of the mind while expelling them into someone else, maintaining contact and control over the other. It is a mechanism for releasing or displacing emotions that are so overwhelming and thus indescribable. Klein thinks that this mechanism exists in everyone, but it expresses a pathological mechanism (Lance, 2011, pp. 101–120). However, Bion argues that Projective Identification can be a positive process; it is an interpersonal experience between two people whose purpose is communication. The unconscious goal is each person's request of the other to experience it.

The object onto which the parts are projected gathers the discarded parts into itself, feels them, and then starts a process aimed at understanding the projected parts, actually changing them in a way that allows their return at a later point. When those parts return to the person, they are different—changed in form and essence. Bion called this process Projective Identification. For Bion, this process, which happens unconsciously, is a communication process (Lance, 2011, pp. 121–140).

In my opinion, the Bionian concept of Projective Identification is central to understanding the motivation and healing processes that occur in the films chosen for this chapter. The directors project outwards parts the Self cannot bear, so that the movie screen will hold the unbearable elements instead of the filmmaker and return the parts of the Self that they *can* handle.

Bion took Klein's original idea of Projective Identification and expanded it into a fundamental understanding of normal development. This development is known as Bion's "containment theory," or "the contained and container." The concept of containment is the ability of one individual to accept the outward projection of another, which he perceives as forms of communication from the other. The receiving object/individual transforms the projection and returns it to the subject in changed form. This process, over time, allows the individual to feel and cope with his emotions and develop his ability to think (Reisenberg-Malcolm, 2008, pp. 220–221). When a person has a container holding his emotions which are then returned after processing, the person learns to think. I thus see the movie as a Bionist container.

The baby's Projective Identification, and the mother who contains her, results in a process of thinking and conversion of mental/psychological elements. Bion calls the patients raw feelings *beta components*. The beta components can only be emitted; they cannot be thought out. The mother (or caregiver) transcends the baby's (or patient's) raw sensations and feelings, in order to transform them into things that in the end she will be able to assimilate into her inner world and use them as components for further development. They therefore return as *alpha components*. When the baby/patient absorbs the alpha components, she can use them as the foundation for her emotional and intellectual development (Reisenberg-Malcolm, 2008, pp. 227–228). That is, thinking is done there. Neville and Joan Symington write that "thinking is a shift from images and ideas a formless state, which are scattered and chaotic (PS state of mind) to a state of coherence and a new understanding is recognized (state D)" (Symington & Symington, 2000, p. 106).

The contents of a movie which deals with sexual abuse are the transformation of beta components into alpha components. The director throws difficult experiences at the screen so they can return to him in a way that he can process and think about them. Bion explains what a thought process is. The thinking process is mentalization: providing symbols for inner experiences. The trauma researchers say that in addition to thinking, it is necessary to build an orderly personal narrative (discussed above). Donald Winnicott, taking a different approach, proposes the creative element of play as a healing modality.

4   Cinema, Therapy, and Donald Winnicott: Play, the Potential Space, Omnipotence, and Holding

Winnicott, like Bion, argued that interpretation was not the main therapeutic tool. Changes in analysis occur when traumatic factors enter psychoanalytic material according to the patient's own path and within the patient's omnipotence range (Winnicott, 2010b, p. 181). It follows that the director can only make a movie following his own path and within his own range. For Winnicott, the therapeutic factor is the patient's ability to play (in the Winnicottian sense) with his or her subjective experience.

Therapy through Play

Winnicott viewed play as a means of achieving psychological health, as the primary tool through which a person can self-actualize and as the nucleus of real life. Winnicott saw play as an act of creation/art (Perroni, 2002, p. 85). Play is fundamentally creative. It should be noted that Winnicott is not talking about the creativity in art, but rather about existing in the world to create.

Winnicott says that creative apperception is what makes a person, more than anything else, feel that life is worth living. Play, in his opinion, helps self-discovery. Communication is only possible during play. The whole human experience is built on the foundation of play (Perroni, 2002, p. 85). For our purposes, a film is an artistic-cultural-media event. Even if the initial association we have with the word *play* is a children's game, Winnicott means every creative action in the world, and the ability to access a subject from different angles and directions, feel it, and think about it. Producing a movie is Winnicottian 'play'; at every stage of the movie, there is playfulness, but the play culminates in the editing stage. A person works scene by scene, changes the order, adds music, adds a new scene before and after the previous one, deletes something, etc. The editing stage allows him to sense and think through the personal story in various forms and ways, until the film takes its final shape.

The Potential Space: The Phenomenon of Transformation

Another novelty of Winnicott is the concept of transitional phenomena: the game the patient plays in the treatment room is not an expression of something internal only, and it does not happen outside of the person, but in the potential space. There, between the interior and the exterior, a person can invent, play, and create (Winnicott, 2010a, pp. 35–56). Winnicott said there are three spaces in one's life experience: the external reality experience that is objective and shared by everyone; the inner reality experience that is mainly subjective; and another reality experience that combines the inside and outside. Winnicott decided to call this third experience "the potential space." A person during her life finds herself in the space that connects the two worlds. In this space, one can actualize the self and the creativity found within.

Rachel Zoran, a bibliotherapist, refers to the phenomenon of Winnicott's transition or transitional object, calling it "the potential space of the artistic experience" (Zoran, 2009). The literary or cinematic text is one of the manifestations of the transitional object or phenomenon, and is referred to as the third part, place, or voice. This is the place for interconnections, a new space between the outside and the inside.

Omnipotence

Winnicott writes that the baby does not acknowledge the fact that the world exists, but thinks that it is he who creates it (Winnicott, 2010a, pp. 35–56). Winnicott assumed that the baby felt omnipotent: the baby's initial feeling was that he is the "king of the world," which he created himself. The baby has the illusion that he is at one with the mother, and it gives him the feeling that he created everything, the whole world. The person who preserves the initial sense of creating the world is a healthy person who can create. Producing a film is an act of creating a world from nothing, and therefore, during the creation process itself, according to Winnicott, healing takes place.

Holding

Holding refers to the mother's or parent's ability to adapt themselves and their care to the baby's developmental processes. As far as Winnicott is concerned, we are always dependent on our object, even as adults. It's a relationship that nourishes us and is important to us. A person does not exist in a vacuum; even when a young person leaves the house they grew up in, they remain somewhat dependent on this connection.

When a mother takes care of her baby, she also physically holds her. This holding is physical possession, but also therapeutic psychological/mental holding, closely monitored and tailored to the baby's needs. This holding lasts an entire lifetime, except that its nature or qualities change. Winnicott wrote that a holder-mother later becomes a supportive environment. For a person to grow into his or her authentic Self, he must live in a facilitating environment. In my mind, the production crew, working on the film, and the abstract idea of "soon I will have a movie," are a replacement for the holding mother. The film itself in all its stages is also holding.

5   Ogden: The Dream Space and the Analytic Third

Ogden, like Bion, talks about dreaming and the dream as a positive thing. Ogden's idea of dreaming is analogous to Bion's thinking. Ogden describes the pathology as an inability to dream, an inability to think about the experience (Ogden, 2013, pp. 216–235). The essence of psychoanalysis, according to Ogden, is to think about the initial and unprocessed experience, to dream the nightmares and the terrors, and to dream and to experience very raw parts. The concept of Ogden's dream can be confusing, because it is actually about the ability to think. According to Ogden's theory, the ability to think is the ability to verbalize a story, make connections between things, and convert impressions into a story (Ogden, 2013, pp. 162–184). This chapter talks about transforming impressions into a movie. Producing a movie is an experience that encourages dreaming which is actually thinking, according to the theories of Ogden and Bion.

Ogden coined a term known as *the analytic third*. There is a therapist and there is a patient, and a third entity is created. That is, the therapist and the therapy are not a place for problem-solving, and the therapist is not an all-knowing authority. Rather, the treatment is a collaborative, reciprocal, and creative process that grows out of the intersubjective space between the subject who is the patient and the subject who is the therapist. It is in this space that a joint creation of this specific, analytical pair is formed (Ogden, 2013, pp. 66–71). The therapist is the one who connects, who translates this intersubjective experience into words. I contend that the film, because it requires translating the filmmaker's experiences into words, represents Ogden's analytic third, as well as Winnicott's potential space.

6 Visibility as a Therapeutic Tool

Jacques Lacan

The viewing phase of the raw material contains another therapeutic element—the visibility. Visibility is complex: the person is seen by others, and she watches herself on screen. It is a developmental stage in which the subject is always trapped, confined to her image. The mirror stage describes the formation of the self through the process of identification with the reflected image. According to French psychoanalyst Jacques Lacan, this initial identification with the image appearing in the mirror is what creates the self. That moment, in which the subject adopts the image as her own, is a moment of supreme joy, thanks to the sense of imagined ownership. The mirror stage is closely related to narcissism (Evans, 2005, pp. 231–232).

I see cinema as a space that contains the Lacanian mirror stage, where a person realizes that he is a singular entity. Or perhaps, his sense of identity is created, along with a sense of joy. Lacan wrote that the reflection of the self in the mirror brings with it a desire to succeed; it is as if that person sees a successful replica of himself in the mirror. The mirror stage is a moment of literal reflection that shapes and defines one's consciousness, thereby shaping the Self. It is a moment of establishing identity while at the same time identifying with the perfect or idealized figure of oneself. Through Lacan, we learn that when we watch ourselves consciously, we feel a desire to improve and succeed.

Heinz Kohut

Austrian psychoanalyst Heinz Kohut wrote about the Self as a psychological entity that organizes a culmination of a variety of experiences. The Self is the center of our actions toward the world; the self is the core of our personality. It reflects the structural characteristics of the personality as well as the resilience for different situations in life at various stages of development. The Self is created and supported through constant interactions between itself and the environment. A healthy developmental process allows the creation of a cohesive sense of self that is consistent over time.

The Self is continuous in that it has a sense of inner harmony, continuity, and unification, but it can also be fragmented, broken, and shattered. The concept of self-object development occurs through the development of a self-object relationship. Self-object is defined as a character or an object that is experienced as part of the self, and its purpose is to support psychological functions that are essential for it. Parents are the first and most central self-objects the child experiences in his early years, and they heavily determine how he is able to internalize other positive self-experiences throughout life.

According to Kohut, throughout our life we need others to strengthen our sense of self. A healthy Self grows through three types of self-objects:

1   **Mirror Axis** (mirroring) (the self-object reflects to the child how wonderful, special, and omnipotent the child is). The joy and happiness that the child receives through the eyes of her parents confirms her initial feelings of power and vitality.
2   **The Axis of Idealization** (the self-object allows the child to see himself as "larger than life," admirable). The child views his parents as powerful, so that he can strive to be like them and receive from them a sense of security and inner peace.
3   **Twinning** (allowing the child to feel a sense of belonging and similarity). Experimenting with a self-object gives the child a sense of imagination and equality, allowing an affiliation to a certain community.

The person who manages to formulate all three of these components in his or her life is a healthy and resilient person, which Kohut refers to as "the Tripolar Self" (Kohut, 2005).

The image reflected in the movie, I believe, constitutes a "self object." The film's narrative takes a compassionate viewpoint that confirms the director's feelings (the Mirror Axis). The character portrayed on screen in the cinema is viewed as a great figure and worthy of admiration. Thus, the hero has new experiences of himself: instead of a victim, he is a revered figure (the axis of idealization). The character portrayed in the movie is similar to the character outside of the movie. The character is similar to the person in real life, and therefore the film's hero has a self-object experience through Twinning (the similarity axis).

The documentaries contain a view of the Self on screen, enabling the Self to feel astonished. The director harnesses the natural power of self-love for healing. Ruth Netzer (2013) adds that in cinema, the narcissistic gaze is transformed into a truth-seeking gaze and self-awareness (p. 24).

Eva Titus

Visibility through the cinema is expanded and intensified further than through the mirror. The psychologist Eva E. Titus argues that video is one of the most powerful tools for changing one's perception of reality. Titus describes the effect caused by the person watching herself in the video (for our purposes, there is no difference between the video and the cinema). According to her, research has shown that the video attracts a lot of attention and shows the viewer a more realistic view of herself, relative to other mediums. The effect of the video is very strong: Titus references a study that showed when psychotic people watched themselves on video, it solicited a new perception of reality. The video uses the patient's narcissistic self-love but redirects it so that the person directs his or her energy outward, into the world. Titus explains how the video differs from a non-video self-image:

- The video takes 25 pictures per second. To see the image, it scans through 625 lines, from left to right on the screen. These are very fast processes that give us the illusion of continuous motion.
- We actually give birth to the picture. We create the picture, and we are involved in building it because of that limitation.
- The video changes the inversion that we are used to when watching ourselves in the mirror. The inversion of gazing at ourselves in the mirror, which we are unconsciously used to, is reversed again. This process is also unconscious. New possibilities open up for the person watching, due to the fact that man does not see himself in the way he is accustomed to. He experiences, sees, and perceives himself differently than he normally would.

Some define treatment as changing how the patient perceives herself. Video causes that shift in perception. In this chapter, we discuss how watching oneself on screen is enough to shift the patient's point of view, even if it is an unconscious change. In this case, a person is actively generating a picture of herself, but *this* picture is different from the self-image she is used to. This version of Self, in the new image, causes a change in her self-perception. Titus references studies that prove a connection between a person's Self-Image, their Self-Concept, and their Exterior Behavior (Titus, 1980, pp. 341–344).

7   Treatment through Group Dynamics

Heinrich Fox

Heinrich Fox, a theorist on group instruction, says that since most of a person's activities are done in a group, psychotherapy should also be done in a group. The group is the most significant agent of change. Humans are inherently social creatures not meant to live in solitude. Within a group, individuality expresses itself as a personal variation on a shared foundation. Because of this, individuality is supported by the group. The individual is part of a social network. An isolated person is like a fish out of water. The framework around the individual shapes his or her experience and values.

According to Fox, illness occurs within a group. Neurotic or psychotic problems are always created within a network of interpersonal relationships and never within the individual when he is isolated. Fox's patient is the one who is isolated from the group. The patient's rehabilitation is his return to a group, and he must find a group to which he belongs.

In this chapter, the film directors are people who have been hurt by other people. Their traumatic experiences isolated them from their communities. The production of the film allows the directors to reconnect with others and form relationships. During the film production, it is assumed that the director bonds with the production crew. A human connection based on the testimony and documentation of the tragedy forms out of empathy, containment, and acceptance. This relationship is further developed into a human connection with the audience.

Irvin Yalom

American psychiatrist Irvin D. Yalom describes the benefits of working within a group:

- Instilling hope (having more hope when part of a society or group)
- A sense of universality (a feeling that I am not alone and there are other people like me)
- Transferring and imparting information (team members pass information from one to the other, from technical to very deep things)
- Mutual help (processes of acceptance and giving) and altruism
- Restoration of the initial family group
- Development of socialization techniques, imitation, interpersonal learning, and group cohesion
- Also, a group provides many points of reference, which creates an environment that encourages higher awareness

(Yalom and Leszcz, 2006, pp. 21–130)

The main concept Yalom emphasizes is group cohesion. Cohesion is the process that connects the group members to each other. In one-on-one therapy, a good therapeutic relationship is an indispensable condition for an effective therapeutic outcome; cohesion is the group therapy equivalent. Yalom says that the concept of cohesion is like the concept of "self-respect"; it can be recognized by anyone, but it seems impossible to accurately describe the concept and certainly impossible to measure it. Yalom describes cohesion as the gravity felt by members of the group: "Coherent group members feel warmth and comfort in the group and a sense of belonging; they value the group and feel they are valued, accepted and supported by the other members" (Yalom and Leszcz, 2006, 72–80). My assumption is that group cohesion is very powerful within the production crew working on the film together. Creating a movie is an exciting event that unites those who are engaged in the craft of making it.

The therapeutic modalities that are listed thus far are relevant for processing any trauma, not just trauma from sexual injury. However, cinema as a medium offers a very powerful solution to problems found only or mainly in sexual trauma, including the paradox of recovery, the need for revenge, and the attack on hope.

8   Cinema's Solutions for Healing from Sexual Trauma

One of the most difficult internal conflicts of sexual abuse victims is the willingness to heal and move on. This involves at least a partial compromise of the victim's identity, letting go of their grip on their anger, and the desire to become a legacy of the harm done.

The Recovery Paradox

The victim fears that if he recovers, heals, and moves on, he is implying that nothing really happened or that what had happened was not so severe, which releases the offender and the people around him from their guilt and accountability. There is an unconscious worry that if the victim heals, it represents how the victim has forgiven or stopped wanting revenge, which is simply not true for many sexual assault victims. Many victims, especially after many years of denial or detachment, have built their identity around the assault. Supposedly, the assault defines the abused, and therefore the possibility of healing stimulates anxiety: If I am not a victim, then who am I? The victim does not know how to build a new identity that is not related directly to the injury, and on which basis he can build that identity (Yael Schvide, lecture, January 31, 2019).

The film gives a very impressive solution to the paradox inherent in recovery. The filmmaker depicts, on screen, that she is actually a victim. She describes what happened and therefore cannot hold on to the thought that if she heals, it is if as nothing happened. The film memorializes the victim identity for the creator so the victim can be released from that identity. The film preserves the victim's narrative instead of the victim preserving it herself. Instead of the victim's life becoming a legacy of the abuse, the film is the commemoration and can build a new identity which is neither part of the victim nor perpetuating the trauma.

The Need for Revenge

Sometimes, *the need for revenge* is the thing that freezes the victim in a static state and does not enable him to heal (Yael Schvide, lecture, January 31, 2019). A documentary film may provide the healthiest possibility for a victim of sexual abuse to cope with the need for revenge, because the film itself is revenge; he accuses the offender out in the open, for the public to bear witness.

The Attack on Hope

Victims of sexual assault face a great deal of difficulty on their way to recovery. Many patients unconsciously experience the so-called *attack on hope*. The patient does not make room to hope, does not believe in hope; they have an unconscious agenda to attack hope. They start healing from a place of despair and disbelief. For many victims, the person/figure who was supposed to keep them safe was the one who hurt them. In traditional therapy, a patient arrives with the thought (conscious or not) that he can be harmed during the therapy as well. Many patients assume that having hope opens them up to disappointment and pain; thus, they want to prove the meaninglessness of the therapist's words.

Victims of sexual assault fear or refuse to let go of the trauma. There is a strong apprehension of the feeling that "everything is fine," because if everything is fine, people will not know and will not understand how much it hurts. A large part of the damage for trauma victims is that others did not acknowledge their pain. A cinematic movie about the sexual trauma is a very impressive solution to the fear of erasing the harm by letting it go. The director shows the world his pain—his wound; he cries out, and, the testimony is on record. Now there is a movie that depicts the testimony, and the movie can always be viewed. The film exists. The director can release the pain and heal, because there is recorded evidence of his pain.

I suggest that the lengthy film creation process slowly loosens the director's grip on the trauma, developing a readiness for recovery. Producing a personal movie causes a shift in the perspective for the director from the position of victim to one of survivor. Since the director is actively creating, she is also the creator of the healing process; she cannot allow herself to devalue the process she is experiencing. She cannot prove the emptiness of the therapist's words because she is the one who creates the words.

Summary: Recovery

So far, we have reviewed the therapeutic factors that exist in creating a documentary film that describes the trauma of childhood sexual abuse. Judith Lewis Herman proposes that recovering from a trauma of sexual injury has three stages:

A Creating security

B Remembrance and mourning: Herman quotes Lipton as finding that unresolved or imperfect mourning leads to stagnation and being trapped in the traumatic process (Herman, 2011, p. 92)

C A renewed relationship with normal life

Herman writes that empowering trauma victims is only possible when the victims are the instigators and masters of their own recovery. The decision to create a film about the trauma is an experience that initiates healing, an event that the director controls, governs, supervises, and directs.

When the directors decided to make a movie and sought out the professionals they would work with (producer, cinematographer, sound person, editor, maybe even researcher, or a lawyer), they created a safety net around themselves. In addition to that safety net, I propose that the camera is a tool that absorbs everything, a tool that receives everything without criticism and judgment. Additionally, the camera is a tool of self-defense: you stand behind it and feel protected. Sometimes the camera can be used as a weapon, if you point the camera at the person who caused the injury.

Thus, the decision to make a movie, finding the people who will work with you and the understanding (possibly unconscious) of the ability to heal while producing the film, is the creation of the director's safety net, which is the first stage of healing.

Working on the film allows the second stage of healing to happen and to recall what happened, and to process it and mourn. The film production phase contains all the therapeutic modalities mentioned. The director gives testimony of what happened, he builds a precise narrative, he plays, and he is the creator of his own world, in which he can dream, think, understand, process, cry, and mourn what happened. After all, he does this not within himself but in the potential space between himself and the outer world. The film becomes an anchor of control; the film holds the director and contains him.

Herman observes that the core of the psychological trauma experience is the disempowerment and disconnection from others, and thus recovery is based on empowerment of the survivor and the creation of new connections. Recovery can only take place within the context of relationships, in which the trauma victim recreates the psychological faculties which were damaged or deformed by the traumatic experience. These faculties include basic capacities for trust, autonomy, initiative, competence, identity, and intimacy (Herman, 2011, p. 163). The film's director works closely with a tight-knit group. Within this team, the director has the opportunity to redevelop social skills which may have been damaged (such as intimacy and trust).

But, when work on the film is over and it is screened for wide audiences, the director allows herself to experience and experiment with the third phase of therapeutic healing: getting back to normal life. At this point, the director stops being the victim of tragic circumstances; she has returned to society as a filmmaker, a creator, with all of the notoriety and praise surrounding this title.

The healing process that happens when producing a documentary does not end with the production of the film, however; it continues during the phase of distributing the film to audiences and conducting conversations with audience members after screening the movie.

Herman (2011) explains how significant the community is in the therapeutic process for the victim's recovery, noting that sharing one's traumatic experience with others allows members of the community to help repair the damage by first declaring publicly that someone in their midst suffered harm, and then by taking responsibility to address the injury through collective action. Through this process, community makes final resolution of the victim's situation possible and also restores the victim's sense of justice and order. While the community viewing the film cannot fix the damage and distortion, it does, however, acknowledge them. In my view, that is good enough.

References

Bell, D. (2008). Projective identification. In C. Bronstein (Ed.), *Kleinian theory: A contemporary perspective* (pp. 174–199). Bookworm Ltd (Tolaat Sfarim).

Caruth, C. (1996). *Unclaimed experience, trauma, narrative and history*. Johns Hopkins University Press.

Deshe, Y. (2017). Living to tell or telling to live. In O. Eshel and Z. Seligman (Eds.), *Haya oh lo haya? (Was it or was it not – When shadows of sexual assault in children appear in therapy)* (pp. 68–100). Carmel Publishing House.

Evans, D. (2005). *An introductory dictionary of Lacanian psychoanalysis*. Resling.

Felman, S., & Laub, D. (2008). *Testimony: Crises of witnessing in literature, psychoanalysis and history*. Resling.

Herman, J. L. (2011). *Trauma and recovery*. Am Oved Publishing.

Kohut, H. (2005). *How does analysis cure?* Am Oved.

Lance, O. (2011). *Psyche introseption* (Hebrew ed.). Amazya Publishing.

Lev-Muhrberg, K. (Director), & Feinro, A. (Producer). (1998). *The diamond inside (HaYahalom SheBefnim)* [Documentary Film]. 52 minutes. https://www.imdb.com/title/tt0171224/?ref_=nm_ov_bio_lk1

Malchiodi, C. A. (2011). *Handbook of art therapy* (2nd ed.) Guilford Press.

Netzer, R. (2013). *The cinema is taking care of us: Patient-practitioner relationships in movies* (Hebrew ed.). Resling.

Nichols, B. (2001). *Introduction to documentary*. Indiana University Press. http://personal.psu.edu/kns5319/ARCH%20130/Bill%20Nichols%20-%20%20Introduction%20to%20documentary.pdf

Ogden, T. H. (2013). *On not being able to dream* (Hebrew ed.). *International Journal of Psychoanalysis*. Psychoanalysis Series.

Perroni, E. (2002). *Acting: A look from psychoanalysis and another place*. Yediot Aharonot.

Rabinowitz, P. (1994). *They must be represented: The politics of documentary*. Verso.

Reisenberg-Malcolm, R. (2008). Bion's theory of containment. In C. Bronstein (Ed.). *Kleinian theory: A contemporary perspective* (pp. 220–238). Bookworm Ltd (Tolaat Sfarim). https://micpp.org/files/psychoanalysis/fargione-primitive-mental-states/Riesenberg-Malcolm-Bions-Theory-of-Containment.pdf

Renov, M. (Ed.). (1993). *Theorizing documentary*. Routledge.

Roth, M. (Director). (2012), & Ofer, R. (Producer). *Pursued (Raduf)* [Documentary Film]. In Yiddish and Hebrew with English subtitles. 51 minutes. https://www.ruthfilms.com/pursued.html

Scherer, Y. (Director), Noy, D., & Ivry, Y. (Producers). (2012). *Dirty laundry (Kvisa Meluchlechet)* [Documentary Film]. 52 minutes. https://www.imdb.com/title/tt5934962/W

Symington, N., & Symington, J. (2000). *The clinical thinking of Wilfred Bion (Makers of modern psychotherapy)* (Hebrew ed.). Bookworm Ltd (Tolaat Sfarim).

Titus, E. E. (1980). Video-feedback in psychotherapy. *Instructional Science*, 9(4), 341–353.

Tuval-Mashiach, R., & Patton, B. (2019). Filming a story: Video-therapy in trauma victims of military background. In Y. Lahav & Z. Solomon (Eds.), *From reliving to remembering: Treatments for trauma* (pp. 233–261). Resling.

Winnicott, D. W. (2010a). *Playing and reality* (Hebrew ed.). Am Oved.

Winnicott, D. W. (2010b). *The true and the false self* (Hebrew ed.). Am Oved.

Yalom, I. D., & Leszcz, M. (2006). *The theory and practice of group psychotherapy* (5th ed.). Kinneret Publishing House.

Zoran, R. (2009). *The letter's imprint: Reading and identity within the bibliotherapeutic dialogue*. Carmel Publishing House.

Index

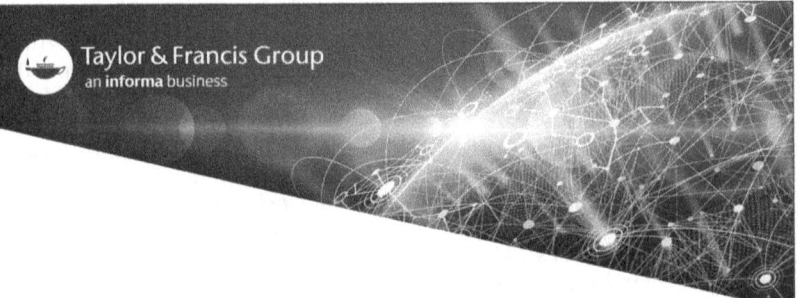
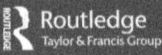
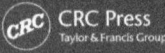